BALANCE AND TREAT THIS HIDDEN ILLNESS
KNOW AND SOLVE THYROID PROBLEMS

THE HOMOEOPATHIC AND THE NATURAL WAY

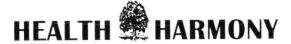

> Note from the Publishers
>
> *Any information given in this book is not intended to be taken as a replacement for medical advice. Any person with a condition requiring medical attention should consult a qualified practitioner or therapeutist.*

KNOW AND SOLVE THYROID PROBLEMS

First Edition: 2004

No part of this book may be reproduced, stored in a retrieval system or transmitted, in any form or by any means, mechanical, photocopying, recording or otherwise, without any prior written permission of the publisher.

© All rights are reserved with the publisher

Price: Rs. 95.00

Published by Kuldeep Jain for

HEALTH 🍁 HARMONY
an imprint of **B. Jain Publishers (P) Ltd.**
1921, Street No. 10, Chuna Mandi,
Paharganj, New Delhi 110 055 (INDIA)
Phones: 2358 0800, 2358 1100, 2358 1300, 2358 3100
Fax: 011-2358 0471; *Email:* bjain@vsnl.com
Website: www.bjainbooks.com

Printed in India by
J.J. Offset Printers
522, FIE, Patpar Ganj, Delhi - 110 092
Phones: 2216 9633, 2215 6128

ISBN: 81-8056-471-1
BOOK CODE: BD-5755

Dedication

Dedicated to my father, Late Shri Hira Nand Dua, my mother, Late Mrs. Savitri Devi, who taught me about the values of life, simplicity, love, compassion and humility and whose guidance inspired me to learn and achieve the goal of my life, the creative writing and Homoeopathy. This book is also dedicated to my brother-in-law, Late Shri Bhushan Lal Arora who all through his simple life inspired me to serve humanity through Homoeopathy on charitable basis.

Dr. Shiv Dua

ABOUT THE AUTHOR

Dr. Shiv Dua, M.A., D.I.Hom., HMD (London) is a known name in the literary world of Homoeopathy. His two books, 'Practitioners Guide to Gallbladder and Kidney Stone' and 'Oral Diseases' have been published. His contribution of homoeopathic articles to magazines like 'The Homoeopathic Heritage,' 'Vital Informer' and 'Homoeopathy for All' is a continuous flow. At present, he is a Medical Officer at Arya Samaj Charitable Hospital, Sector 19, Faridabad where he conducts his daily service to patients.

Contents

Section 1

The Endocrine System 1
Thyroid Gland Diseases 31
Goiter 43
Hypothyroidism Myxedema 71
Hyperthyroidism— Thyrotoxicosis 103
Therapeutic Suggestions 135
Differential Diagnosis of Swelling of the Neck 143

Section 2

Alternative Therapies 151

Section 3

Thyroid Function Tests 173
Importance of Thyroid Function Tests 189
Role of Homoeopathy 195
Should Allopathic Medicine be Stopped 223
Is There any Prevention? 231
Last word 241
Bibliography 242

ACKNOWLEDGEMENTS

I wish to acknowledge the following individuals whose efforts have contributed to the creation of this book:

Dr. R.S. Chandans, Ex-President, HMAI Faridabad unit for his support and commitment to homoeopathy.

Dr. Sanjeev Kumar, Gerneral Secretary, HMAI, Faridabad unit for his continuous encouragement to me in writing this book.

Dr. Jitender Singh, President, HMAI, Faridabad unit for his inspiration and valuable comments during the proceeding of the monthly scientific meetings.

Dr. Lalit Aggrawal, Member, Council of System of Homoeopathic Medicines, Haryana and Vice President, HMAI, Faridabad unit.

Uma, Dharmesh, Amit, Nilima and Anu for their whole heartedly cooperation in preparing and revising the manuscript of the book.

N.D. Nagpal, P.L. Rawl, J.D. Rawl, Himanshu Arora, Lalita, Kailash, Krishna and Usha for their inspiration to me from time to time in writing this book.

Akshay, Tanya and Dipesh, the kids, whose curiosity did not tempt them to bother me during my serious work sessions in my computer room for completing this book.

Dr. Shiv Dua

INTRODUCTION

It is amazing that we live in a world of computers and electronics, having most advanced gadgets of life to serve us and yet we know little about our own bodies. We know far more about the latest inventions but do not know what goes on beneath the skin of our body. The subject of our education in a particular field say engineering, teaching, accountancy or any other field making us earn our living is satisfying but beyond the subject we are taught in, very few of us know about the functions of our body. We go to a doctor and then know about the name of disease. Beyond this, we do not desire to know except taking the prescribed medicines. If we know our body well, the whole set up of thinking of a man changes especially in respect to disease he suffers from. One must have an idea as to which system of medicine has limitations and which system can give long-term relief. Besides this, one should also know what are the things or eatables to be avoided in each disease and which are the things to be taken during the disease so that the effects of the disease are reduced.

We do not know the endocrine system of our body and one of them is about the role of glands, especially the thyroid gland, which is in the major part of the body, the neck. It is the neck, which holds this wonderful and useful gland known as thyroid.

This gland is the generator of our body and if it is diseased, under-active or over-active, swollen or painful, it will bring in several initial disorders which are not easily diagnosed till a doctor advises the blood tests. The facility for testing thyroid functions is not easily available in small towns and villages. This is the greatest handicap and most of the people deprived of this test take wrong medicines of debility, anemia etc., which in turn aggravates the condition of thyroid.

SOME FACTS

- People in India are not aware that nuclear fall out is one of the causes for thyroid diseases. Conducting an open-air nuclear bomb test is supposed to throw the inhabitants of the area to thyroid diseases. This has been proved. *Chernobyl's nuclear disaster* produced biggest group of thyroid cancer. Almost 2000 confirmed cases of thyroid cancer have resulted from 1986 accident-cases and almost 5 million faced increased cancer risk (A report of the American Association of Thyroid). Thyroid health problem still plagues the Ukraine and other areas that were downwind of world's worst disasters.

- There is still another surprise that people are not aware that the disease has its origin from hereditary aspects. *The American Association of Endocrinologists reveal that more than 3/4th (76%) of the population of America do not know that thyroid disease runs in families.*

- Research in USA also shows that millions of thyroid patients are undiagnosed. A strong link has been found *between autoimmunity and thyroid disease.*

- Some researchers have found out that the major cause of illness is the *food-borne bacteria,* which can contribute to or even trigger autoimmune diseases connected with thyroid.

- Researchers of USA have formulated another amazing theory and according to this, each person has his or her own 'normal' thyroid function and it is known as 'normal' in the report of the laboratory but *this does not necessarily mean that thyroid is normal.*

- The fear of thyroid diseases is so alarming that people in USA and European countries have purchased preventive pills from the market. According to the experts there, Potassium iodide pills (KIO_3 TM) can protect the thyroid against damage from certain nuclear accidents or a terrorist attack on nuclear establishments. The Americans are so sensitive that after the arrest of alleged 'Al Qaida members' on 10th June 2002, the cost of the above pill has skyrocketed.

There are some diseases where the doctor of the conventional system prescribes continuous *medication* throughout one's life and this can trigger a patient to get more depressed or worried about one's health. The diseases like hypertension, diabetes and disorders of thyroid are some examples in which life-long continued medication is prescribed. People in general know about high blood pressure and diabetes, being very common diseases, but are not aware of the functions and disorders of thyroid-related diseases. Thyroid-related diseases like hyperthyroidism and hypothyroidism have hidden illnesses, the symptoms of which are not identified in the first instance.

This attempt of writing on the subject should make it easy to identify the disease on clearer frame. This disease is common in women or should we say that it affects women frequently than men.

What is thyroid and what are its functions in our body is the basic question everyone would like to know first?

Our body is full of wonderful organs knitted into such a beautiful network that even the minutest cell of the body cannot survive without the help of its neighbouring tissue, cell or organ. A complete unit of human body is something no scientist can ever dream of creating. We can never fully understand the functions of our internal organs. Had it been so, the mankind might have invented the methods of longevity and would never fall sick. We may boast and declare that we know the actual functioning of each of the organs of the body but can never know its complete identity. Blissfully, homoeopathy does not believe in depending upon the exclusive knowledge of an organ to find out the cause of its non-functioning. It does not conduct experiments of drugs on animals to record results. All experiments of drugs are made on human beings in homeopathy. People having normal health are induced with the drugs and the symptoms produced by the drug on such healthy persons are recorded. This is how the *law of similars* is put into action. *The symptoms produced by the drug and the symptoms in ailing body produces should be a similar in all respects. This type of 'like cures like' principle is what we call Homoeopathy.* The name of the disease has no meaning for homoeopaths. This principle is very much applicable in the case of persons suffering from thyroid problems. As I said, the patients suffering from thyroid disease do not know in the first instance as to what is the name of disease they are suffering from. Even when a doctor of the allopathic system of medicine is consulted, he encounters doubts. To have a clear idea of the disease, he refers the case to the clinical laboratories before making a final verdict. On the other hand, if the patient happens to consult a homoeopath, the symptoms of the disease would lead to the remedy and clear the case within a definite span of period. Naming the disease is of no concern to the homoeopath. This book has been written for the general public and layman, so that he is aware of this gland. One knows about the heart, liver, intestines, spine, brain, kidneys and even gall bladder but thyroid has a distant occupancy of functioning in the body. One fine morning, after the laboratory tests are declared, the doctor tells the patient about the thyroid problem. The patient is taken aback as to what is this thyroid about? Now the patient is at the mercy of the doctor. The prescription is made and handed over to the patient. More of the annoyance is that the patient is advised not to miss a tablet for even a single day throughout his life till the doctor advises. It is at this stage that the patient needs guidance. The book will help him/her to know what he/she did not know about this disease. The patient can thus manage the disease and decide the next line of treatment or discontinuation of drugs. Naturally, it will be switching over to the homeopathic way, changes in diet and life style and conducting Yoga besides other excercises.

During our practice, we meet many patients who come to the homoeopaths for suggestion of an alternative to the daily intake of pill prescribed for thyroid problems. In about ninety five percent of cases reported to me, I have found that they did not even know the existence of thyroid gland in the body? Some people know that it is some organ related with the throat and its function is to produce hormones. Beyond this, the conventional doctors treating the patients do not detail anything. The purpose of the book is to explain the functioning of the thyroid gland, its diseases and conditions under which the disease can be eradicated by homoeopathy and natural way. The book's intention is to display the mysteries of the thyroid clearly and exhibit rational solutions. The readers may feel worthy to complement the sheer magnificance of the structure and working of human body, a God's creation. The fascinating hidden world of this wonderful gland will surely interest the readers because every effort has been made to resort to a simple narration that can be easily understood by a layman and the students of homoeopathy.

Date: 11.03.2003

Dr. Shiv Dua

SECTION - 1

The Endocrine System

ENDOCRINE GLANDS

Most of our body functions are governed and guided by endocrine glands to maintain a harmony between all body organs. These endocrine glands secrete some chemicals called *hormones* into our blood stream. Through the circulation of blood in the body, the messages of the brain are carried and relayed to different organs so as to enable them to undertake the specific processes like growth of the body and reproduction. Hormones are chiefly connected with metabolism of the body and their intention is to make an interaction among the organs to achieve the desired results. In other words, we can say that *hormones are chemical messengers of the body*. These hormones are produced by glands situated in different parts of the body wherefrom these are released or circulated in the blood to the body cells, which need them and which can be called as targets. These target cells make an effect after being provided with the hormones. The glands which are responsible for producing and releasing the hormones of the body are the collection of ductless or endocrine glands. These so-called endocrine glands release their products directly into the blood and not through a tube or duct as exocrine glands do. Hormones are slow workers and take much longer time to act or we can say that hormones tend to act slowly and produce their activity over a considerably delayed period, the example of which can be seen in growth and reproduction. Besides growth and reproduction, their basic job is concerned with controlling or affecting the chemistry of the cells on which they target. The target cells in turn affect the rate of consuming food substances and releasing energy in tune with the quantity and quality of the hormones released. Hormones have widely spread effects.

Thyroid gland is one of the ten glands that make up the endocrine or hormonal system. We shall have to understand many aspects and activities of various glands before thyroid is explained.

The beauty of the glands is that secretion exists but they are without excretory ducts. Their production is a special substance called hormones—a word, which is derived from Greek word *hormao* which means excite. The secretion of the glands is directly into the blood. Throughout the human organism, the hormones are delivered and the process of this delivery either stimulates or depresses the receiving organ. This fluctuation or disturbance of hormone supply can bring about changes in the body. The changes increasing the functions of the gland are termed as *hyperfunction* and the changes decreasing the functions of the gland are termed as *hypofunction*. In other words, secretion of a superfluous quantity of hormones by a gland of hormones is called hyperfunctioning and secreting insufficient amount of hormones is called hypofunctioning. The supply of hormones measures fraction of milligram in 24 hours. Actually, the hormones are imbedded with very high biological activity. The endocrine glands include thyroid, parathyroid, epiphysis cerebro (pineal), pituitary, thymus, pancreas, adrenal and gonads (sex glands). These glands are glandular epithelial tissues which have extensive accumulation of blood vessels and nerve fibers. They form a collective system themselves and are interconnected. The glands are regulated by the nervous system, which exercises direct control over the endocrine glands by dint of nerves and neurohumoral control. The effect of hormones is through the blood and this is called *humoral regulation*. The pituitary gland or hypophysis cerebro is the main gland of the endocrine system, which produces special substances to stimulate the activities of the other glands, and has a special reference with thyroid gland. Before we take up the connection of pituitary gland with that of thyroid, we ought to know the role of hormones.

HORMONES—HOW THEY WORK?

There are various chemical reactions going on in the body. There have to be chemical messengers and *they are called hormones*. The hormones are manufactured by our endocrine glands located in different parts of the body and the hormones always travel through blood and act upon different body cells, which we can call as targets of hormones. It is these targets which are affected. If we compare hormones with nerves, we find that the hormones are slow pacers. They act slowly and take a longer time to achieve the required result. Hormones have a tendency to control and influence the chemistry of the *target cells*. It is the hormones which determine the rate at which they use up the food material and then release energy. It is also the job of hormones to determine whether there should be milk production (females) or hair growth or body growth, and if so at which rate the metabolic processes should act? There are some general hormones made by main endocrine glands. *Two examples are sex hormones and insulin*. There are other hormones, which act very near to the point of production and one of them is local hormone *secretin*, which is made in the duodenum and it is secreted in response to the presence of incoming food. It is a wonderful combination when the same hormone travels to a short distance in the blood to reach the pancreas for stimulating it so that there is a flood of juice (*enzymes* or chemical transformers). It is these enzymes or juice, which are very essential for digestion. Similarly there is another local hormone called *acetylcholine*, which is made every time a nerve conveys a message to a muscle cell for contraction. Such is the wonderful history of hormones about which still more is to be learned. There has been a continuous research work on this, which is still going on.

PROTEINS & STEROIDS IN HORMONES

In our body, almost all the hormones are quite active but in very small quantity. A very small amount of hormone is needed, in some cases, to carry out a specific task of the concerned organ. It may be even less than a millionth of a gram which accomplishes the target.

There are two varieties of hormones. One, which are *protein based or are derivatives of protein* and the second, which have *structure like a ring or a steroid*. Our main concern in this book is thyroid and we must know that *thyroid hormones are prepared from a protein* base and are protein derivatives. *Insulin is a protein hormone.* On the other hand, the *sex hormones* and hormones manufactured by the cortex or outer part of the *adrenal gland are both steroid hormones*.

HOW A HORMONE WORKS?

The working of the hormone is subject to a proper place and environment of the surrounding of the organ. Upon reaching of the hormone in the area of its target, it goes on the job only if it finds itself in a rightly and correctly shaped site on the target cell membrane. After the hormone finds itself locked in the receptor cell or site, it does its work by stimulating the formation of a substance named *cyclic adenosine monophosphate or AMP*. The cyclic AMP is supposed to do its job by stimulating a chain of enzyme system within the area of a cell. This limitation is due to the fact that all specified reactions should stimulate and make the required product, it is supposed to transform. What function it has to target, depends upon the assignment given to the hormone by its producer.

For example, *cyclic AMP manufactured by the presence of insulin hormone prompts the cells to take up and use glucose.* On the other hand, the hormone *glucagon* made by pancreatic gland compels the cells to release glucose, which in turn is used in the blood as energy giving stimulant, known best for physical activity. We must appreciate the amazing working of hormones. *Once the hormones have done their job in a particular area of work, they become inactive or* in some cases carried to the liver for making it inactive. The liver breaks them down to make new hormone molecules or simply converts them for excretion.

EMOTIONS & HORMONE LEVELS

Our body is a strong bridge of links. There are links and links between each and every part of the body and continuity is a must to make it an entity called human being. Hormones have direct links with acts of our daily routine jobs and the part they play in displaying our emotions is vital. If a mother is waiting for her son to return and when the son does not turn up at the time he was to come, the mother gets upset and in many mothers it is to the effect that emotional upset becomes physical. They may report frequent stools, vomiting and so on. There is a link between the pituitary gland and the brain and it has a direct and definite connection between hormones and emotions. Another example of such a change of hormonal aspects upon the emotions can be witnessed—If a woman is worried and under great tension for some reason or the other, her menstrual cycle timings may be altered. The tensions can change the level of hormones like estrogen and progesterone. It is these hormones, which control the periods. Some women unnecessarily worry too much about their date of periods and such tensions are known as premenstrual symptoms, and such an act is due to sudden fall of hormone levels. On the other hand, if the level of hormones is high in the mid-cycle, it is supposed to be good and women feels a sense of well-being.

Actually, this is the time when the women give good response to sexual acts and are most fertile as well. If the women at this juncture of mid-cycle are worried and under tension, such emotional factors can change or alter the hormone levels.

Emotions play a greater part in the sexual acts. The level of estrogen and progesterone hormones generally rise during the sexual foreplay because of direct handling leading to pleasurable impulses on the brain. If the husband taking part in the sexual act does not play in accordance with the choice of wife or if there is a repulsive partner, the whole act is simply a turn-off and hormone production is inhibited.

Similarly, the emotions play havoc after the reproductive life of a woman come to an end or when menopause approaches. There is a lot of emotional disturbance and this is due to lack of response to follicle stimulating hormones by the ovaries and there is total stoppage to the manufacture of estrogen and progesterone. Not only that the hormones are partly withdrawn but also there is evidence that most of this behavior is psychological. The same type of menopausal emotional upsets occur when a woman gives birth to a baby. In this case also, there is a withdrawal of sex hormones from the body, which is temporary but emotional effects have almost a similarity with those of women who undergo the steady process of menopause.

PRIMARY HORMONES & THEIR FUNCTIONS

Growth hormones	Regulates the growth of body.
Prolactin	Responsible for milk production.
Oxytocin	Initiates the process of labor.
Antidiuretic	Maintains the water level in the body.
Thyroid	Keeps the whole of body system active.
Parathyroid	Maintains blood calcium level.

Adrenals	Produce adrenalin to prepare body for action.
Cortisone	Manages stress level.
Aldosterone	It controls the body's salt level.
Pancreas	Insulin maintains the blood sugar level.
Estrogen and progesterone	Maintains and controls the menstruation and pregnancy.
Testosterone	Controls the male sexual characteristics.

HYPOTHALAMUS

Hypothalamus is one of the most important groups of cells in the body, which is on job 24 hours a day. Its prime job is to maintain equilibrium inside the body and inform the regions of the brain and body for their action. *If thyroid has been termed as generator of the body, hypothalamus is its main switch.* It is a sort of coordinator between the pituitary gland and the nervous system of the body.

Hypothalamus is located underside the brain, just near the center of the head. It is almost pink and gray in color and has a size of a small prune (dried plum) weighing about 1/300 of the mass of brain. On account of its dealing with developing a sensing system and direct or indirect nerve connection, it has a far more richer blood supply than other parts of the body.

Hypothalamus has a wonderful capacity in preparing the body in extremes of temperature be it minus 50° F or 120° F and the amazing part of the job is that body temperature remains normal i.e. 98.4° F. In a condition when the body goes hot during extreme rise of temperature in summer, it is this gland, which sends message to the pituitary gland. Through the sympathetic nervous system, the message is conveyed to the tissues to dilate the surface blood vessels and open sweat glands. Naturally, the sweat glands cool the skin and the body gets rid of the high temperature of the climate. Similarly, at the same time, the hypothalamus sends message to the brain to speed up breathing so that gasping or long yearning is started to carry away the heat. On the other hand, if there is extreme cold and fall of temperature, hypothalamus sends message to the adrenal and pituitary glands for release of more of blood sugar from the liver so that such type of fuel for muscles warm up the body. Hypothalamus is also responsible for causing shivering of the body. Shivering will naturally produce heat in the body by friction. Sweat glands also shut down and the skin muscles get tightened and the hair on the skin stand up. All this is a sort of insulation against the cold. *Hypothalamus, therefore, works as a thermostat.* Irrespective of the temperature outside the body, hypothalamus maintains the temperature inside. There is very little and rare that goes wrong with this gland because it is well protected and not prone to injuries. Of course, tumors can affect the surroundings of the gland thus impeding the blood supply to the brain.

Besides, the hypothalamus also manages the water balance in the body. [When the blood grows too salty due to lack of water, ADH is released through joint effort of hypothalamus and pituitary. This additional ADH enables the kidneys to absorb more water than usual with the result that urine is concentrated and salivary glands reduce their flow of saliva. This means that body will conserve all the water it has, and the person will feel thirsty. Drinking more water will now balance the water in the body and blood will be no more extra salty. Take another example, if the blood becomes more watery after taking a lot of cold drinks, beer, etc., the hypothalamus sends a message to the pituitary to reduce the amount of ADH release in the blood stream. With this step, kidneys will not conserve water at the usual rate and work fast to produce urine at a faster rate so that extra water is thrown out.]

Hypothalamus is one of the links between the endocrine glands and the nervous system of our body. It has a main function to convey and relay impulses and work as a stimuli between the brain and the organs located far from the brain. For example, kidney-link and brain-link is processed by hypothalamus. When we talk of links, there is a link between the nerve cells of the hypothalamus and the secretions of the anterior part of the pituitary gland. When the nerve cells of the brain release some chemical transmitter substance, the hypothalamus receives it and in response to this sort of a trigger, it releases the hormones. We have example of ADH (antidiuretic hormone) and oxytocin hormones. These are manufactured by the pituitary gland under the direct control of nerve impulses made by the hypothalamus and are released by the pituitary. Special nerve cells in the hypothalamus accomplish this releasing task and they act on the cells of the anterior pituitary before they release their hormones.

PITUITARY GLAND (HYPOPHYSIS)

GENERAL

Pituitary gland plays a key role in the body. Its powerful hormones can create wonder or havoc in the body. A perfect normal existence is possible if the gland is working perfectly and if it is not working normally, it can sicken the body with a bizarre spectrum of diseases or even kill the body. It is one of the hormones of the pituitary gland, which gives a push to the baby in the world. It is again the pituitary hormones, which decide the size of a body—a dwarf, a giant or a normal; hastens the ageing process of the body. On the other hand, it can shrink the size or sexual organs of a man back to boy-size. It is the job of the pituitary gland to monitor the activity of other glands and to check that they produce the right amount of hormones. In short, it can be called the *chemical boss of the body. It is a tiny 'chemical plant' in the body*. The pituitary gland produces about ten hormones, the substances of which are complex. The total daily output of these hormones is less than 1/1,000,000 of a gram.

THE MEDICAL POINT OF VIEW

Pituitary gland is a very small body, pinkish in colour, oval in shape, and pea-size nubbin of tissue and weighs about 0.5 gm, 85 percent of which is water. It hangs like a cherry, on a tiny stem from the underside of the brain. It is the master gland of the body. It rests comfortably inside a protective body, a bony saddle called *sella turcica*. [Sella turcica is a Latin word meaning 'turkish saddle] Sella turcica can be easily visualized in the X-ray of the skull (in case, enlargement of the sella is seen in the X-ray, the disorder of the pituitary gland can not be ruled out; the other tests should be conducted.). Pituitary gland is so much protected that no head injury from outside can harm it until directly pierced with some sharp arm. If the pituitary gland is injured, the result on the body will be dramatic. It is situated in the cranial cavity and is connected with hypothalamus. Hypothalamus is a region of the brain, which is joined to the pituitary by a short stalk of nerve fibers. It is the work of the hypothalamus to coordinate the function of the nerves and endocrine system of the body. Hypothalamus is concerned with the production of two hormones as described above under hypothalamus. Pituitary gland has an *anterior lobe,* a *middle part* and a *posterior lobe* and their borders can be seen only with the help of a microscope. The anterior pituitary has no direct path of nerves to connect it to the hypothalamus. Pituitary has to bank upon a series of special releasing or restricting factors to control the release of hormones. These factors (some of them) are specialized hormones, which are released by hypothalamus and act upon the pituitary gland situated a few millimeters away. The pituitary portal system has a special set of blood cells meant to carry the hormones and this system runs between the pituitary and the hypothalamus. The anterior lobe produces many hormones like *somatotropic, thyrotropic, adrenocorticotropic (ACTH) and gonadotropic.* The functions of *somatotropic* is related with growth of the body, and influences metabolism particularly synthesis of proteins in the tissues. *Thyrotropic hormone* affects the thyroid gland. The *adrenocorticotropic* stimulates the function of the adrenal glands and *gonadotropic* hormone stimulates the sex glands. Gonadotropic has two branches of hormones called FSH (follicle stimulating hormones) and LH (luteinizing hormones). The sex glands stimulate the production of two major sex hormones, *estrogen and progesterone*. In the females, these two hormones control the menstrual cycle whereas in the males, FSH and LH stimulate the production of male hormones and sperms.

The dysfunction of the anterior lobe of the pituitary gland brings in many changes related to growth.

In childhood, if the secretion of this lobe is excessive than required rate, the result is *gigantism*. Those who are affected by this may reach a height of 2.5 meters or above because excessive secretion means excessive growth of the bones of face, fingers and toes with enlarged nose, tongue and other organs. Such a disease is called *acromegaly*. On the other hand, if the secretion is less from the lobe, the result is retarded growth i.e. *dwarfism*.

Growth hormones have another important job to do in our daily routine life. Even if someone is fifty years of age and if he breaks his bone in an accident or cuts his face with his razor by mistake, it is believed that growth hormone hasten the process of healing. The growth hormone might be inciting growth of new tissue to replace the worn or torn out tissues.

The posterior lobe of this gland secretes *oxytocin and vasopressin*. Role of oxytocin in the body is not very clear. Oxytocin is supposed to stimulate the contractions of the uterine muscles and is used to boost weak labor. It also plays a vital role in starting the secretion of milk from the breasts during lactation. Oxytocin, in males has a different role. It is supposed to be connected with generation of orgasm. As a matter of fact, the anterior pituitary also releases hormone *prolactin*, which appears to act directly on the tissues without stimulating some other gland. Prolactin is very much connected with controlling the means of reproduction and has a complicated role to play in females than in males. The role it plays in the males is not very clear but it is determined that excess of prolactin can have ill effects on male's health. In the females, the prolactin stimulates the breasts to produce milk. *When the milk is present in large amount in the breasts, it inhibits ovulation and the menstrual cycle.*

Coming back to *vasopressin*, it actually makes the contraction of the blood vessels of the uterus. In vasopressin, there is lack of antidiuretic hormone (ADH), which makes the blood to absorb water into the blood on the higher side. ADH is concerned with the control of water in the body. It acts on the tubules of the kidneys affecting their ability to retain or release water. When ADH is secreted into the blood, the kidneys conserve the water and when ADH is not released, more water is released from the body in the form of urine. *Hypofunction* of this posterior lobe of the pituitary gland causes a decrease in the secretion of the antidiuretic hormone. Naturally, such a disturbance in the water metabolism results in *diabetes insipidus*. We shall not discuss much about this disease except that it is characterized by intense thirst and passing large quantity of urine. Some experts claim that the hormones secreted by the posterior lobe of the pituitary are not produced by it but by the nerve nuclei of the hypothalamus and then are deposited in the posterior lobe [Injury of the gland may result into a dramatic situation. It lowers the production of ADH, which actually controls the urine making in the kidneys. In the event of injury, the kidneys would produce heavy quantum of urine, perhaps many liters a day.].

We shall not go into the details or functions of other glands of the body and take their reference as and when the topic suggests. One must keep in mind that like all the glands in the body, *the thyroid gland is under the direct control of pituitary gland.*

SUMMARY OF THE HORMONAL ACTIVITY OF THE PITUITARY

TSH	Stimulates the thyroid gland to produce thyroid hormone.
ACTH	Stimulates adrenal glands to produce cortisone.
Oxytocin	Meant for initiating the labor process and breast milk.
ADH	It controls the balance of water in the body.
FSH and LH	Responsible for production of estrogen, progesterone and testosterone (sex hormones).
Prolactin	Causes breast milk production.
Growth Hormones	Controls growth of the body.

INTERACTION BETWEEN THE PITUITARY & THYROID

It is in very simple terms and you can understand it fully. When the level of thyroid hormone is low, the pituitary gland secrets thyroid stimulating hormone (TSH), which sets off its production. When the quantity of thyroid hormone is sufficient, the pituitary gland stops producing TSH. A complete harmony is maintained between the two till both the organs are in good working order.

PARATHYROID GLANDS

The parathyroids are the four small oval bodies, located behind the thyroid glands (posterior surface of the thyroid gland). Two of them can be called superior and two are inferior. Each of them weighs about 0.5 gms. Although the functions of parathyroid glands is not very clear yet an outline describes their job. They undertake a major part in controlling the levels of calcium in the body. A hormone called *parathormone* has been isolated from these glands. Parathormone produced by parathyroid is a polypeptide with a molecular weight of 8600 (Rasmussen). Both calcium and phosphorus metabolism in the organism is influenced by these glands. Bones and the kidneys are the chief target organs. Calcium and phosphate are mobilized from the bones by direct action. The kidneys excrete phosphate. There is reciprocity between phosphate and calcium. If these glands are removed from the body, there will be sharp decrease of calcium in the blood plasma. Such a condition is called *tetany* and this results in intense spasm of the muscles. Without removal of the glands, if such a condition exists (spasms of muscles), it is the hypofunction of parathyroid. Tetany is, therefore, responsible for the disturbance of calcium metabolism in children. It leads to tooth decay. It affects the pregnant women. Such conditions can be misjudged by the doctor as lack of vitamin D. Calcium is a very essential component of the body and this mineral helps in building the structural element in the formation of bones and teeth besides its major role in the activation of muscles and nerve cells. We know that the calcium level of the body has to be maintained with a fair constant boundary, the failure of which may cause the stoppage of working of the muscle. *The parathyroid glands keep the calcium level in constant balance.*

We have already discussed about the production of calcitonin. We know that parafollicular cells of the thyroid produce this hormone, which is responsible for regulating the calcium levels of the body. Calcium also manufactures the bones besides triggering impulses in the nerves and muscle cells to maintain the calcium level in the blood. As a matter of fact, calcium coordinates and acts with another hormone, parathormone (PTH). *Parathyroid, the four tiny glands located behind the thyroid gland* produce PTH. PTH raises the blood level of calcium whenever the body needs calcium by stimulating the release of calcium from the bones. Stimulation is done by increasing the reabsorption of calcium from the kidneys and converting vitamin D into a hormone, which increases the gut reabsorption of calcium. In this way, the calcium level is increased and once it is accomplished, the thyroid releases calcitonin, which suppresses the release of further calcium from the bone.

The parathyroids are very small and tiny and it is very difficult to locate them. The upper two are situated behind the thyroid gland and the two lower ones are inside the thyroid.

THE THYROID GLAND

The primary function of thyroid gland is to regulate the metabolism of the body. The diseases of thyroid, either hyper or hypothyroidism is 'term-wise' well known in America where more than five million Americans have this common medical condition. About ten percent of women may have some degree of thyroid hormone disturbance, i.e., either over production or deficiency. As a matter of fact, millions of people suffer from it and they do not know that they have some thyroid problem till the condition is aggravated. The treatment of many thyroid conditions warrants surgical removal of a part or whole of the thyroid gland. If the total mass of thyroid-producing cells within the body is not sufficient to the demand of body, the patient may develop *hypothyroidism*. In severe conditions only when cancer is suspected, thyroid gland is removed surgically or a part of it is removed. The remaining part (lobe and isthmus) can produce enough hormones to meet the demands of the body in some patients. Some patients have conditions that can be treated with *radioactive iodine therapy*. The aim here is also the same, i.e., to kill a portion of thyroid to prevent goiters from growing larger or producing too much hormones. This condition is *hyperthyroidism*.

In America, (or possibly in India), video-assisted thyroid removal is possible. Such an operation leaves a scar of less than one inch even when the complete thyroid gland is removed.

In the later part of the book, we shall discuss about the main reasons for hypothyroidism and hyperthyroidism.

Where do we see the thyroid gland in the body? Well, we do not see it when it is in its normal position. This grand gland moves during the act of our swallowing food or liquid together with the larynx and its slightest enlargement during the course of any disorder exhibits its presence. It can be then inspected by palpation. Thyroid gland is pinkish in color, butterfly shaped and it straddles the windpipe just below the Adam's apple. *In case you are in the prime of your age and slim, you may be able to find the outline of your thyroid gland. Stretch your neck and look into the mirror and try to swallow your saliva. Now you may be able to see the gland moving up and down.* If you are obese with thick neck, you may be able to feel it moving by touch of your fingers during the act of swallowing. Even if you are unable to see or feel it by the touch of your finger, do not get upset. Many of us cannot feel or touch. In case of enlargement of this gland due to some reason, the voice changes and marked enlargement of the gland leads to difficult breathing due to the fact that both trachea and larynx are compressed. In some diseases, the thyroid does not move during the act of swallowing. In such cases it may be localized partly or completely behind the sternum and compress the adjacent vessels. You must have seen the enlargement of thyroid during the act of swallowing both in persons who are healthy and diseased. The most comforting part of any disease of thyroid gland is that it is not life threatening although it is a source of debility, tiredness, depression and discomfort in the initial stages.

The thyroid gland develops in the body from the very first week of life near the root of the tongue. It is then a small piece of tissue. At the time of growing of the unborn baby, the piece of this tissue at the root of the tongue moves down to the neck through a narrow passage (thyroglossal duct) and settles at the place where adults have it. When the baby or foetus is about three months old, this gland starts working.

LOCATION

Thyroid gland is located in the anterior surface of the neck just below the level of larynx. It is a soft gland, small in size weighing about 15 to 25 gms (There is a variation in the weight in the view of some experts and they claim that it is 30 to 60 gms.). In adults it is almost 20 gms. Its hormone production is less than 1/2,2800,000 grams in a day. Although *thyroid is small, say around the size of a plum,* yet it has a tremendous responsibility to carry out amazing jobs of bodily processes. In our ancient medical books, it has been considered vital to life. In Hindus when they die and are cremated, the remains of the bones called 'phool' are handed over to the kith and kin of the dead for further disposal in the sacred rivers. In north India, the 'pandit' performing the last rites takes out a bone piece to show you and calls it 'Atma ram' or soul. This is nothing but the bone remains of thyroid cartilage (Adam's apple). We cannot live without thyroid gland although the medical science claims that one can live without it provided a regular artificial replacement of thyroid hormones are inducted to the body which is practically not possible.

Thyroid can be compared with the bellows of blacksmiths. It fans the fire of life controlling the rate at which billions of cells burn food into energy. Either it banks the fire or fans it into raging flames. If it produces too little of hormones, the person becomes obese, sluggish, obese and dull. If it is over productive in hormones, the person has canine appetite but will be rail-thin due to burning up of his food at a rapid rate. The patient's eye would pop to an extent that he would not be able to close his lids over them. *In a nut shell, thyroid gland is a tiny chemical plant, selecting materials from the bloodstream and fitting them together to make complex hormones.* Its two major hormones are approximately two-third of iodine, and the requirement of iodine is about 1/5000 gram. Iodine comes from the digestive tract in the form of iodide. Enzymes convert iodide into iodine and then hook this iodine to an amino acid (tyrosine) within the body. After conversion, two chief hormones are formed. Again enzymes come in the picture to hook molecules of these hormones to blood proteins and carry it to the remotest corners of the body.

The power of the hormones thus produced is tremendous but it has to be kept under control and fed to the body needing exact energy at any given moment. If a lady is pregnant, she would require slightly more hormones than usual to meet her needs. If the person sleeps, his requirement of energy is minimum but when he gets up or there is slightest activity, the need of hormones differs. Two other glands, hypothalamus and the pituitary maintain the necessary control of hormone production.

PHYSIOLOGY OF THE THYROID GLAND

There are *two lobes in the thyroid gland*, which lie in front and either side of the trachea as it passes down the form of neck, which means that it is asymmetrical to the larynx and trachea. The right lobe is nearer to the surface and the *left lobe* is bounded by the larynx and trachea on one side and esophagus on the other. The two lobes are joined by a small connection or bridge of tissue, which can be called *isthmus*. Sometimes, the isthmus gives off a *pyramidal lobe*, which extends upwards. The thyroid gland has a number of vesicles or follicles with walls of glandular epithelium. The cavities of the vesicles are full of colloid, viscous substance possibly secreted by the lining cells. This colloid contains *thyroxine* and *tri-iodothyronine*, the hormones of the thyroid gland. They possess iodine. As the length of name indicates, tri-iodothyronine is several times more active than thyroxine. These hormones make an impact on the metabolism concerning the growth and development of the organism and excitability of the nervous system.

The main function of the gland is to produce *thyroxine and tri-iodothyronine* (T4 and T3) hormones. *Thyroxine* contains about 67 percent of iodine and a shortage of this element diminishes its production. Daily need of the body for thyroxine is between half and one milligram. The functional activity of the normal gland differs at different times of the year and there is variation in the iodine contents. All the hormones of thyroid control the heart and metabolic rate besides producing the *calcitonin*, which regulates the concentration of calcium in the blood. The pituitary gland situated in the brain produces *thyroid-stimulating hormone* (TSH), which triggers the flow of thyroxine (T4) from the thyroid.

In short, we can say that thyroid gland produces a chemical called thyrotropin-releasing hormone (TRH) and this triggers the pituitary into secreting the thyroid-stimulating hormone (TSH), which in turn sparks the release of thyroxine (T4) and tri-iodothyronine (T3).

THE ROLE OF HORMONE T3

On the other hand, if we cut down our diet of starchy food, it will decrease metabolism causing the body to produce less of T3. If the thyroid is working properly, it will protect us from starving and keep the body weight more or less stable. Thyroid hormones give us a protective mechanism to overcome period of starvation and overfeeding. It is this wonderful mechanism by which people live even without taking anything for a long time. People starving at sea, on mountains and during the worst disasters of natural calamities like earthquakes covered in the debris of fallen houses are found alive after several days of their retrieval from the trappings. This is the wonder of T3. The suffix of three in T3 is due to its containing three atoms of iodine. We shall know more about the functions of iodine in the following paragraphs.

THE ROLE OF HORMONE T4

In case of shortage of thyroid hormones during pregnancy, there can be lot of havoc. Low level of thyroid hormone T4 has the capability of damaging the development of the unborn baby's brain. This in turn can cause undergrowth of brain and the baby may be born mentally deficient, a condition called *cretinism*. On the other hand, thyroid hormones have the capacity to totally transform the cells to a stage of maturity. The cells of the body pertaining to different organs develop the characteristics of the organs to which they belong. It is this process which makes the embryo to develop from a small cluster of cells to a fully-grown baby. So, besides the formation and determination of the length and strength of the bones, the hormones of the thyroid strengthen the cells of the body. The beauty is that the cells pertaining to a particular field, say intestines, will develop for the purpose they are meant. In the initial stage all the cells of the embryo are same, undifferentiated, but as the embryo starts to grow the cells begin to become specialized in the field they are embedded. Without the induction of T4, this process cannot happen. The suffix of four in T4 is because it has four atoms of iodine in it.

CARRYING OF HORMONES BY T3 AND T4

In its practical application, the job of T3 and T4 is done through carrying around in the blood stream bound in two proteins. The remaining part, a very minute fraction, floats free in the blood. They targets on the particular organ and once they reach their destination, they get released from their protein bindings and surprisingly T4 is converted into the active T3 form, ready for use by the cells. The free-floating T3 is not released from its protein-binding and is available for instant use.

THYROID GLAND AS A GENERATOR OF THE BODY

Thyroid gland can be compared with the generator, which releases energy for whole of the body. Its prime job is to control the metabolism (or the pace of activities or a change) of each cell of our body. The hormones of thyroid activate mitochondria, the tiny cells that produce energy. These cells are actually powerhouse of the energy. It is this energy release, which controls our appetite and temperature. It ensures that the body remains at normal temperature whatever be the temperature of the environment outside, be it extreme cold or extreme hot. It is here that the metabolism of the body is influenced by the hormones of the thyroid. It fixes up the rate at which the cells of the body burn up oxygen. It is a process we are involved within ourselves in everyday life, be it normal breathing, drinking, eating, sleeping, walking around or sitting idle. It is again this process of metabolism of the body influenced by the hormones secreted by the thyroid that our heart beats, the process of digestion takes place, working of the brain takes place and activities of the reproductive organs get stimulated.

GROWTH FACTOR AND THYROID GLAND

Let it be clear that when we talk of reproductive organs, it is again the thyroid, which is involved in the *development of breasts in women*. The mental and physical growth depends upon the activities of hormones produced by thyroid. In coordination with somatotropin (STH), the growth hormone released by the pituitary gland, the working of *thyroid hormones determines the height, length and strength of bones*. Any shortage of thyroid hormones stunts the growth of the body by obstructing the bones from growing and maturing.

The growth hormone is most important during the childhood and adolescence but it has equal importance in the later part of life too because it determines the way the body tissues handle carbohydrates.

ROLE OF VITAMINS AND THYROID GLAND

When we talk of growth, we cannot remain silent on the intake of nutritional food containing balanced intake of vitamins. Why to talk of the efficient working of thyroid gland alone; it is the vitamins, which give total protection to us against all diseases. If vitamin intake is balanced in the body, there is no reason why thyroid gland should not work efficiently. It is all a team-work of all the organs to combine and combat diseases provided they are strong. To keep them strong, vitamins are needed. Let us find out what is the role of vitamins in our body.

Vitamin A is good for skin, eyes, restoring reproductive power and strengthening the body.

Vitamin B1 has effect on appetite, muscles, constipation and fatigue, nervous tension and *thyroid gland*.

Vitamin B2 is good for eyes and skin.

Vitamin B6 has effect on arteries; causes anemia, diarrhea, mental disorders and helps in building up the resistance.

Vitamin B12 is mainly responsible for pernicious anemia.

Vitamin C balances the power of resistance, prevents bleeding from gums and teeth; useful in arthritis and cataract.

Vitamin D is useful in weakness, myopia and rickets besides absorbing calcium and phosphorus in the body.

Vitamin E is useful in controlling the blood pressure, complaints of menses in women, bodyaches, heart diseases, reproductive organs, helps in safety of retina of eye etc.

Vitamins to be taken by thyroid patients

The patients of thyroid diseases mostly suffer from following diseases or disorders and should take the following vitamins in the form of food products or even can take the pills of the mentioned vitamins on the recommendation of a physician.

Associated symptoms/diseases with thyroid gland diseases

Name of disease/disorder/symptom	Vitamin recommended
Emotional disturbance	B6
Fatigue	B1
Gall bladder stone	B6
Kidney stone	A
Menses	E
Anemia	B6 and D
Pernicious anemia	B12
Weakness	D and B6
Constipation	B1
Skin problems	B1 and B2
Appetite	B1
Arthritis	C

HOMOEOPATHY, VITAMINS AND BIOCHEMICS

In the homoeopathic system of medicines there is no theory which prevents the intake of nutritional food and to supplement it by the vitamins. No homoeopath should be averse to vitamin intake by the patient. Along with the intake of vitamins, homoeopathic medicine can be given keeping an interval of atleast half an hour between the two.

As a matter of fact, the human being or human organism works on the system of complete integrated totality following or acting upon the directives of innate intelligence. This intelligence is a cumulative effort of all the systems working in the body and it is this intelligence, which cures the body of diseases.

By presenting the organism strength of both the *vital force agents, (homoeopathy) and vitamins,* the system should react in an affirmative manner. All true sciences—Allopathy, Ayurveda, Unani or Homoeopathy, are interrelated. The ground-work of all the systems is common and thoroughly understood. There should be no objection by the fraternity if vitamins and tonics of other systems are used with homoeopathic remedy. If the homoeopathic remedy is correct according to the law of similars, there is no reason why vitamins should create any hurdle in the process of cure. Doctors, who understand homoeopathy, rarely misunderstand other systems of medicines.

Those who are against the use of vitamins with homoeopathic medicines may use Biochemic medicines. *Schussler*, the scientist doctor responsible for starting a new branch of biochemic medicines and *Hering*, an eminent Homoeopath, were of the opinion that like deficiency of vitamins, lack of tissue remedies (12 elemental substances in the body) can be the cause of many diseases. These elemental substances are biochemical salts, which are present in our food. These can be taken if there is any deficiency of any one or more of them in the body, just like vitamins. These twelve salts are Calcarea fluorica, Calcarea phosphoricum, Calcarea sulphuricum, Ferrum phosphoricum, Kalium phosphoricum, Kalium muriaticum, Kalium sulphuricum, Magnesia phosphoricum, Natrium muriaticum, Natrium phosphoricum, Natrium sulphuricum and Silicea. In accordance with the law of biochemistry, the deficiency of these salts can cause diseases.

It can be said that the basic principle behind the vitamin deficiency and the tissue salt deficiency is the same. If it is so, there is no reason why better results cannot be obtained by the use of vitamins and biochemic salts together. Many eminent homoeopaths are practicing on this principle by giving both homoeopathic medicines and biochemic medicines together.

THYROID GLAND AND ITS CONNECTIONS

Thyroid gland is not only for the existence in the form of a gland to execute certain functions but it has multiple connections. Here we shall discuss about these connection.

Infections and Thyroid Connection

Thyroid has a special role to play for *protection against the infection*. It plays a vital role in the upkeep of our immune defense system. Thyroid has the capacity to stimulate very special cells situated in the lymph nodes. These cells are called T cells, they help the body to fight against the diseases. To fight against the infections, the body has to possess good immune system. Many thyroid diseases are caused by the autoimmunity disorders when the body is unable to identify its own tissues and as a matter of their procedural nature, produce antibodies against them. Diseases like goiter and its associate diseases like Grave's disease (over activity of thyroid) and Hashimoto's disease (under active thyroid) are the result of the same autoimmunity.

Ageing and thyroid connection

Ageing is another phenomenon, which has a direct link with functioning of thyroid. The process of growing is supposed to be triggered by pituitary and thyroid but the possibility of the process of growing older is yet to be ascertained by the research scientists. One aspect has been determined that thyroid's effect on metabolism has some part to play in the ageing. Practically, it has been observed by some scientists that cutting short on food or undereating can slow down the ageing. This means that age linked degenerative diseases of the old persons are linked with food intake. This has been specifically mentioned in our ancient books on medical science i.e. the system of *Ayurveda* that *observing periodical fasts prolong the longevity*. If we can agree that the role of metabolism and hormones is significant enough in harmonizing the body's various functions, we cannot rule out that thyroid has something to do with ageing. Now following the same way of thinking, just visualize about the function of hormones and its connection with the functions of liver. Both thyroid and liver are interlinked.

The hormones of thyroid are supposed to convert beta-carotene into vitamin A. Beta-carotene is a pigment, which induces color to vegetables and fruits. Along with vitamin A, vitamin C and vitamin E make a difference in fighting against degenerative diseases of the old persons. Even cancer and heart ailments may be prevented if the metabolism is sufficiently enriched with above vitamins. If thyroid is in order and its functioning is normal, premature ageing and degenerative diseases should not occur. Ageing has a definite link with thyroid gland.

Vitamin B1 and thyroid connection

It is well known that deficiency of Vitamin B1 (Thiamine) is responsible for disorders like Beri-Beri, anorexia, constipation, bodyache and general fatigue. It is also noted that deficiency of B1 can lead to nervous tension. Deficiency of Thiamine (B1), Pyridoxine (Vitamin B6) and Niacin altogether or separately cause high irritability and restlessness to the extent of mental imbalance.

So far as the connection of vitamin B1 with the thyroid gland is concerned, it is simply understood. If obesity is the outcome of the thyroid disease in a particular case, there is disorder of metabolism in the body for which this gland is responsible. *Dr. Russel Walter of England conducted some experiments on human beings and showed that deficiency of vitamin B1 stops the functioning of thyroid gland.* When this vitamin was restored, the thyroid gland became active again. He made it clear that instead of giving any medicine made of thyroid gland, it is better to give vitamin B1 first to remove weakness. *(Book: From old age to youth through Yoga by Dr. Satyavarta Siddantalankar.)*

When there is goiter or enlargement of neck, the cause is related to thyroid. Thyroid gland becomes weak and it becomes enlarge so that it can discharge the function of metabolism properly and efficiently. Doctors then administer iodine or medicine made out of the thyroid gland.

Induction of vitamin B1 is supposed to be best for helping thyroid to function properly in the views of some doctors.

Vitamin B1 is not present in good quantity in Indian diet. In some fruit juices, it is found in very small quantities. It is mainly found in brewer's yeast and germinated wheat. There is a method to germinate the wheat by keeping its grains (seeds) in water. Gram seeds can also be germinated in the same manner like wheat seeds. *Sago* is supposed to be rich source of vitamin B1. (Sago is a starch). For non-vegetarians, the source of this vitamin is liver part of the meat. The daily requirement of vitamin B1 is about 1.2 to 1.8 milligrams for men and about 1.5 milligrams for women. This vitamin gets destroyed by heat and alkaline products and remains intact when there is acidity in the body. In some cases, this vitamin is not digestible and produces urticaria (skin disease). Patients suffering from urticaria and coming to the doctors for consultations should be particularly enquired as to whether they are taking vitamin B1 either in the form of pills or foodstuff containing liver or germinated grams or wheat, etc. It is advisable that all patients suffering form urticaria should be told not to take vitamin B1 products till the disease is cured.

THE IODINE FACTOR

Another aspect in discussing about thyroid, which we cannot ignore while discussing about ageing, is *iodine* factor. Iodine plays a vital role in producing thyroid hormones. Iodine is a trace element mostly found in the foods like milk, eggs, butter, cream, cheese, spinach, lettuce, peanuts, sea salt and iodized salt, pineapple, meat and fish and some grains and cereals. It is a chemical essential for our body cells to work. Our body has an average of twenty to thirty milligrams of iodine, most of which is concentrated in thyroid. In order to maintain the level of iodine in thyroid, we need to take at least 100 to 200 micrograms of iodine daily from our food. It is the iodine, which combines with other chemicals to make T3 and T4 hormones. If you check with the food items containing iodine, it is sure that everyone of us, vegetarian or non vegetarian, is bound to take grains, cereals, salt and milk or milk products in our daily needs of the diet. Iodine has been an essential component in our diet since time immemorial and we cannot live without taking it in one form or the other. In people living in far-flung hilly areas salt is a precious commodity and is used sparingly. It is always missing in the soil and water. The same is true in the areas, which were once glaciated. Once the glaciers melt, they wash iodine out of soil. The result is that the inhabitants of such areas suffer from *nontoxic or iodine deficient goiter*. It is not an essential reason but a general observation that reduced salt intake (iodine) can cause goiter. We shall discuss about goiter when the diseases of thyroid are explained. In short, non-toxic goiter is due to lack of iodine and it is a sort of swelling in the thyroid gland, easily visible on the front portion of neck. In olden days, people used to apply iodine sponges on the outer surface of neck to get relief from the disease.

Due to some reason, many aspects can trigger overproduction of iodine. In such case, thyroid may enlarge diffusely just as it is when there is shortage of iodine production. This is toxic goiter. Thus, we see that shortage or overproduction of iodine both can cause different types of goiters.

Nervous and Chemical Controls—Its Thyroid Connection

Besides getting help from the hypothalamus and pituitary glands in controlling the activity of thyroid, the thyroid itself controls the nervous and chemical metabolism. Any kind of stress and worry is capable of producing excessive amount of hormones, which are sufficient to affect the brain, leading to mental disorder. For example, if there is some shock to the person in the event of death of some near and dear, a business failure, a serious accident or surgery of some relative of the person, some marital problem, some inconvenient sufferings and over and above, if such problems go on piling one upon the other over a period of months or years, there is likely to be a chain reaction in the brain. Such a condition will make the hypothalamus over-stimulate the pituitary, which in turn over-stimulates the thyroid.

In short, the thyroid is one of the weakest spot in the body so far as emotional turmoil and sentimental shocks are concerned. A great deal can go wrong with its functioning and then the troubles starts physically.

Beauty and Thyroid Connection

In layman's language and not in a professional tune, it is to be noted that secretions from the thyroid gland mix with the blood and keep the body healthy. Remove this gland or make it weaker by partial removal, you will find even a young man of twenty years will show signs of ageing, looking like an old man. There will be premature wrinkles on the face ahead of old age. It has been proved by many experiments conducted by the scientists that thyroid gland has a major role to play in maintaining and retaining youth. As a matter of fact, the work of this gland is to keep the body slim, trim, active and beautiful. Active and slim or beautiful is one who has nails and hair healthy, and whose face is shining and wrinkle free. Some doctors in the western countries call this gland as *Beauty Master*.

Doctors who are connected with the beauty clinics always prescribe medicines made up of this gland for removing obesity, wrinkles and even acne. Whether this type of treatment on the part of managers of beauty parlors is effective or not is not known. One important aspect connecting beauty with thyroid has been observed that some of the facial disorders connected with hormonal imbalance, of which acne is one, are cured by homoeopathic treatment. In case of obstinate acne, *Thyroidinum* 3x has been found quite effective when given under the perfect regime of symptomatic ruling.

■

Thyroid Gland Diseases

THE IMPROPER functioning of thyroid gland leads to many diseases. These are *hyperthyroidism (thyrotoxicosis); hypothyroidism (myxoedema); cretinism (dwarf); goiter (simple, nodular, solitary nodule, retrosternal); toxic goiter (diffuse toxic, toxic nodular, toxic nodule); tumors of thyroid gland, infections of thyroid gland, thyrioditis (granulomatous and autoimmune) and many other diseases connected with hyperthyroidism and hypothyroidism like cardiac rhythm disorder, myopathic, and retinal myxoedema.* Besides these, there are diseases of the thyroid gland with thyroglossal duct too.

GENERAL EXAMINATION

Within our trachea, there are ring-like structures. At the level of second to fourth such ring rests the normal thyroid gland. It is on either side of the midline of the tracheal rings. The two lateral lobes of thyroid lie along the lower half of the lateral margin of the thyroid cartilage. Each lobe measures 5 cm in length, 3 cm in width and 2 cm in thickness.

VISUAL OBSERVATIONS

Thick layer on the neck

When you check the gland, it will not be observed in its normal position. The patient will have a short neck, will be obese, has myxoedema or has scleroderma.

Position of the gland looks abnormal

If you feel that the position of the thyroid is abnormal, there is likelihood of following conditions:

(i) Displacement of the gland.

(ii) Ectopic thyroid.

(iii) Absence of thyroid gland.

Displacement of the gland
Lateral

If the displacement of gland appears lateral, there are three possibilities:

(a) Malignant lymph nodes.

(b) Sternomastoid tumor.

(c) Carotid and subclavian aneurysms.

Anterior

If the displacement appears anterior, there could be growth in the larynx or even a cold abscess from the cervical spine.

Ectopic thyroid

Some residual thyroid tissue along the course of the thyroglossal tract is common. It may be *lingual, cervical or median* (thyroglossal). It is rare that whole of the gland is ecotopic.

Lingual thyroid

It can be seen at the back of the tongue at the foramen caecum. It forms a round swelling there. Due to this condition, the patient may find difficulty or impairment in speech, dysphagia and respiratory obstruction.

Median ectopic

Thyroid forms a swelling on the upper part of the neck and is usually mistaken as thyroglossal cyst.

Cervical Ectopic

Cervical (lateral aberrant thyroid) lumps on side of the neck side are uncommon. There is no evidence that aberrant thyroid tissue occurs in the lateral position. Normal thyroid tissues are separate from the thyroid gland and should be treated as metastasis in the cervical lymph node from an occult thyroid carcinoma.

Absence of the gland

Such a condition should be enquired from the patient before setting in for examination. Either the absence of the gland is *congenital* or the patient had undergone *thyroidectomy*.

Check the Skin Over the Gland

The skin over the gland is generally normal in look but may have following features as well in some cases:

- If the skin is smooth and dry, the possibility is myxoedema.
- If the skin is smooth but has excessive sweating, it is thyrotoxicosis.
- If the skin has slight dusky-blue discoloration, it is a large goiter or a hemorrhagic goiter.
- If the skin appears red, the case is that of acute thyroiditis or the patient has been recently treated by radio-iodine therapy.

Examination of the Swelling on the Neck Area

Swelling on the neck has to be examined in particular manner, searching the area and the location of the swelling. One has to know the different places of the neck to confirm the different situations of the swelling.

First, note the condition of the skin over it. There may be redness, edema, presence of subcutaneous dilated veins etc. Sometimes, it is observed that the skin is stuck down at one spot on the swelling, which in turn causes a fold of the skin to stand out below it. This is a characteristic feature of malignant growth such as secondary carcinoma in lymph nodes.

Also examine, if there is a sinus, fistula, ulcer or a scar in the area. Tuberculous sinus or ulcer generally seen is due to outbursting of caseous lymph nodes and this is quite common in the neck. In some patients, there is a transverse linear scar seen. This looks exactly like an incisional scar resulting from the healing of several tuberculous sinuses or ulcers. Sinus due to *osteomyelitis* of the mandible is usually single and lies a little below the jaw. If there are multiple sinuses over an indurate mass at the upper part of the neck, this indicates *actinomycosis*, for which one should look for sulphur-like grains in the pus. If there is a *gummatous ulcer* in the sternomastoid muscle, it is rare. About *bronchial fistula*, its favourite site is the lower third of the anterior border of the sternomastoid muscle.

Where can the swelling, cysts and fistula occur?

- The swelling can be over the area of parotid gland. The area is on the inner side of the outer ear, towards the direction of lips.
- Swelling can be on the submaxillary salivary gland area, below the jaws.
- It can be on the bronchial cyst area, which is the area below the parotid gland.
- It can be on the sternomastoid muscle, which is on the posterior part of the bronchial cyst area or the surrounding area of bronchial cyst.

- It can be on the carotid body situated behind the bifurcation of the common carotid artery or below the bronchial cyst area.
- It can be on the thyroglossal cyst, which is the area of thyroid, moving up and down when swallowing.
- It can be on the area of bronchial fistula and area below thyroglossal tract.

Check the Veins Over the Neck
- If the veins over the neck are prominent and distended, *thyrotoxicosis* is the possibility.
- If the veins over the neck are dilated and tortuous, *retrosternal goiter* cannot be ruled out.

Check the Enlargement of the Gland
- The enlargement seen on the gland may be due to normal functional activity (*a colloid goiter*), decreased functional activity (*thyroiditis*) or increased functional activity (*Grave's disease*).
- If the enlargement is sudden, the possibility of hemorrhage in the thyroid swelling exists.
- If the enlargement is gradual, there may be increased vascularity (*thyrotoxicosis*), increased epithelial cells (*colloid goiter*) or increased fibrous tissue (*Hashimoto's disease*).
- If the enlargement is localized, it may be *nodular goiter, a cyst of thyroid, a cystic degeneration or a localized hypertrophy.*
- If the enlargement looks diffuse, it may be *physiological or pathological.* In physiological, the reason is puberty, pregnancy and menstruation. In the absence of physiological reasons, *thyrotoxicosis or Hashimoto's* disease may be concluded.
- If the enlargement is irregular, it may be *multinodular goiter.* In such conditions, *malignancy* cannot be ruled out.

PALPATION

The thyroid gland has to be palpated from front and behind. Ask the patient to keep the neck slightly flexed and undertake the act of swallowing while you are palpating. According to the view of the experts, the thyroid gland or the presence of nodules in its substance can be palpated by simply placing the thumb on the thyroid gland while the patient swallows.

Lahey's method

Palpation of each lobe is best carried out by this method. Let the doctor stand in front of the patient. If the left lobe of the thyroid is to be examined, the thyroid gland is pushed to the left from the right side. It is *vice versa* for the right lobe. The lobes are thus made prominent and palpated with the other hand. During the course of palpation, the doctor has to check the position, the extent, the size and shape of the swelling. Its consistency has to be determined carefully as follows:

If the feel is *rubbery*, the thyroid is *normal*.

If the palpation is *soft*, it may be a *thyroid cyst* or *Grave's disease*.

If the palpation is *soft and elastic*, it is *diffuse colloid goiter*.

If the palpation is *firm*, Hashimoto's disease cannot be ruled out.

If the palpation is *quite hard*, one can assume Riedel's thyroiditis or a *carcinoma*. [Riedel's thyroiditis is very rare in goiters. In this condition, the thyroid tissue is replaced by cellular fibrous tissue, which infiltrates through the capsule into the adjacent muscles, paratracheal connective tissue and carotid sheath. It is a collagen disease and the goiter is unilateral or bilateral, very hard and fixed.]

Mobility

Let the doctor move the swelling of the patient vertically and horizontally and determine the extent of mobility. Check carefully its relation with the neighbouring structures like trachea, esophagus, larynx, recurrent, laryngeal nerve, carotid sheath, and sympathetic trunk, adjoining muscles, skin and subcutaneous tissues. See if swelling displaces the trachea or larynx. A thyroid swelling may compress the trachea from both sides giving rise to what is called a *scabbard trachea*. If there is displacement of the esophagus by a thyroid swelling, the result is dysphagia. A benign swelling of the thyroid gland displaces the carotid sheath backwards where the pulsation of the carotid artery can be felt. On the other hand, a malignant thyroid engulfs the sheath completely so that no pulsation of the artery can be detected.

If there is involvement of the sympathetic trunk, it is *Horner's syndrome*, which means a bit of drooping of upper eyelids, slight sinking of the eyeball into the orbit, contraction of the pupil and absence of sweating on the affected side of the face.

- Put your fingers on the growth and roll sidewise and up-down position for checking the mobility.
- If mobility is *restricted*, it may be *colloid goiter*.
- If the mobility is *absent* altogether, it may be *chronic thyroiditis* or a *carcinoma*.

GENERAL AUSCULTATION AND PERCUSSION

- Percussion can be done over the manubrium sterni to find any increase in the supracardiac dullness in a suspected case of retrosternal goiter. It is seldom helpful.
- A continuous murmur without heart disease suggests thyrotoxicosis. In primary toxic goiter, a systolic bruit may be heard due to increased vascularity.

MEASUREMENT

Measurement of the circumference of the neck is important in goiters because it will give an idea about the increase or decrease in the size of swelling after medication.

GENERAL EXAMINATION

Whenever there is doubt about Hashimoto's disease, it is better to examine the liver and spleen of the patient to see if any cirrhosis exists.

EXAMINATION FOR TOXIC MANIFESTATIONS

In primary goiter or exophthalmos (protrusion of eyeball), one should keep in mind that there are four main features:

1. *Von Graefe's sign:* It is lagging behind of the upper eyelid when the patient is told to look downwards.
2. *Moebius sign:* In it, the convergence of the eyes is found difficult by the patient.
3. *Stellwag's sign:* There will be infrequent winking and also retraction of the upper eyelid.
4. *Joffroy's sign:* When the patient is told to look upwards keeping the face inclined downwards, there will be no wrinkling of the forehead.

When the thyroid gland is enlarged but the enlargement is not evident, this means the gland is slightly enlarged. In such a condition, a *thrill* is frequently palpable due to increased vascularity. On conducting auscultation, a systolic bruit may be heard, when this thyroid-thrill exists. (See general auscultation and percussion above).

Increases pulse rate or tachycardia, that is without any rise in the body temperature is always due to primary toxic goiter. The pulse rate is variable from 90 to 180 per minute.

Examination of the patient to check tremors is equally important. Direct the patient to stretch out his or her arms in such a way that the arms are parallel to the ground. Also tell the patient to spread the fingers. Now check the fingers, which will be showing fine tremors. There is another check also for tremors. Tell the patient to put out the tongue and the doctor can observe fibrillary twitching. In very severe cases, the whole body of the patient is shaky and trembling.

Discussing about *tremors*, it is notable that in *secondary toxic goiter,* exophthalmos and tremors are not marked features and they do not exist. In it, the main effect is on cardiovascular system, where-in, the pulse gradually becomes irregular in rate as well as in rhythm. (Secondary toxic goiter is the toxicity supervening on a long-standing thyroid adenoma or nodular goiter. It is separately explained in the goiter section of the book).

Metastasis is another condition when the thyroid swelling is of hard stony nature and has fixity with irregular feel, it is better to go in for distant metastasis especially in the skull or long bones where there may be a swelling or a pathological fracture.

THYROID NODULES

When the thyroid becomes overactive, it is not only a condition pointing towards Grave's disease but there may be fault in the thyroid gland, which causes it to produce too many hormones thus creating a lumpy swelling. We shall be discussing about this in the chapter on Goiter later. If the goiter exists and the condition is such that the thyroid is overactive, the swelling will become more lumpy and irregular or nodular. We should know that a nodular goiter is mostly caused by shortage or excess of iodine in the diet or by use of certain drugs. Sometimes, it is due to over stimulation of part of the thyroid by TSH, the thyroid hormone produced by the pituitary. There is a thyroid hormone therapy or TSH suppression therapy for thyroid nodules. Let us have a view.

Thyroid Hormone Therapy or TSH Suppression Therapy

[This therapy is not put into practice as a routine for treatment of nodules. As a matter of fact, it is used when there is suspicion of cancerous growth and the patient is not healthy enough to go in for a surgery. This therapy is used when the patient develops thyroid nodules after getting treatment in the form of radiation to the head, neck or chest and also there has been a partial removal of thyroid gland (lobectomy). Also when there had been surgery for thyroid cancer. Thyroid hormone therapy is often given to reduce the TSH in the body, preventing growth of any remaining thyroid cancer cells.]

In this therapy, the patient takes some medicine orally. Theses medicines are Liotrix (thyrolar), Liothyronine sodium (cytomel), Levothyroxine sodium (synthroid, levoxyl, levothroid) and desiccated thyroid (armour thyroid). It is known or believed that the persons having thyroid nodules are normal so far as their thyroid functioning is concerned. This means their thyroid is producing the right amount of thyroid hormones. Now when this additional thyroid hormone in the form of above medicines is introduced to the body, the pituitary gland in the brain detects the excess thyroid hormones and stops making thyroid-stimulating hormones (TSH). This is why this therapy is called *TSH suppression therapy also.* Now when TSH is secreted less, the thyroid gland produces smaller amounts of thyroid hormones, which in turn may stop or decrease the growth of nodules.

FACTS ABOUT THE NODULES

Recently there have been research and studies in Nosulwa in U.S.A., and it was found out that:

- In cases of benign thyroid nodules, it is quite common that they go away without any treatment.
- But this does not mean that the treatment should not be done. It has not been possible to say whether nodules, treated with thyroid hormone, would go away of its own.
- TSH is not the only reason for affecting thyroid nodule growth and hence there is no certainty that lowering TSH level can stop growth of nodule.
- The studies have been made on smaller groups of people and hence no one is sure that thyroid hormone therapy is an accepted scientific method.

Are There Any Side Effects of This Therapy?

- High doses of thyroid hormone can lead to overactive thyroid gland or we can say that hyperthyroidism can develop.
- There may be worse effects of this hormone therapy on people who suffer from heart disease. They may have increased risk of heart attacks (myocardial infarction), heart rhythm irregularities, chest pain or angina.
- Those people who do not keep good health and suffer from minor ailments from time to time may have less serious side effects of this therapy. This includes diarrhea, headache, appetite variation, weight loss, tension, anxiety and irritability.
- It is always better to go in for biopsy of the nodule so that above complications are avoided. If the nodule goes on increasing in size during the therapy, the thyroid hormone therapy should be stopped immediately.

Goiter

AN ENLARGEMENT of the thyroid gland is known as *goiter* in simplest definition. It is the condition in which the entire gland may be swollen or the center or the right or the left lobe only are swollen. The swelling is non-neoplastic and non-inflammatory. The term goiter is derived from Latin word *Gutter,* which means throat. It is a chronic hypertrophy and hyperplasia and there is variation of size. Some goiters are enormous in size. Locality is a prominent cause and it occurs as an epidemic disease in mountain regions. Sporadic cases may be found everywhere. Soil and water are two frequent causes in which either soil or water or both may be rich in lime. Magnesia and calcarea are the two salts responsible in most of the hilly areas. It is also a fact that unhygienic surroundings and weakened constitutions are the predisposing causes. The disease is not infectious as has been demonstrated in recent times.

Whenever you travel to hilly areas, it is common sight to see a person with swollen neck at the front. Villagers do not take the disease seriously and they resort to local medication including applicants. In local language it is called "Galgand," "Ghenga," or "Rasoli". The government has made good publicity by printing and circulating posters in the government hospitals for an awareness of the disease. The poster states that the disease is due to shortage of iodine in the salt and government advises the public to use iodized salt.

WORLD HEALTH ORGANIZATION ON IODINE DEFICIENCY DISORDERS

Goiter is iodine deficiency disorder. It is a deficiency that affects the central nervous system and this disorder is found in every continent of the world. The WHO has chalked out a program to conquer this disease in all continents by the year 2010 at a projected cost of 75 million dollars. According to this report, close to 1.5 billion people have iodine-poor diets, which can afflict entire population with reduced intellectual capacity, impaired motor functions or *goiter*. The strategy for conquering this disease is relatively simple; add iodine to salt and get people to use it. The iodination program is relatively inexpensive but must be maintained permanently. (Courtesy SPAN)

CLASSIFICATION OF GOITERS

GOITER (SIMPLE)

A simple goiter is endemic or sporadic and it may be either a diffused hyperplastic goiter or a nodular goiter.

A simple goiter is also called physiological goiter or puberty goiter.

TOXIC GOITER (THYROTOXICOSIS OR HYPERTHYROIDISM)

Toxic, as the meaning of the word suggests, is the bacterial poison in blood. Toxic does not mean excessive secretion of hormones but toxic symptoms develop due to hyperthyroidism.

NEOPLASTIC GOITER

Neoplastic goiter may be malignant or benign.

Benign is true solid adenoma (Fetal cell or papillary and Hurthel cell adenoma).

Malignant is in three forms:

(i) *Primary carcinoma*

Papillary, alveolar, anaplastic and medullar.

(ii) *Secondary carcinoma*

(iii) *Lymphoma*

Reticulum cell sarcoma, lymphosarcoma.

THYROIDITIS

Thyroiditis is the inflammation of thyroid gland. It may be granulomatous or autoimmune.

Thyroiditis can be classified into three varieties:

(i) Granulomatous thyroiditis.

(ii) Autoimmune thyroditis-Lympth adenoid goiter-Hashimoto's disease.

(iii) Acute bacterial thyroiditis.

RARE GOITERS

Chronic bacterial thyroiditis, acute bacterial thyroiditis and amyloidal goiter are three rare types of goiters.

SIMPLE GOITER (BRONCHOCELE)

The prime reason for this type of simple goiter is on account of stimulation of the thyroid gland by the anterior pituitary. In this state, low levels of circulating thyroid hormones increase the TSH secretion. Leave aside TSH, any reason, which leads to persistent low level of circulation thyroid hormones can be a cause of simple goiter. Any reason means first of its kind as *deficiency of iodine*. The daily requirement of iodine is about 100-125 mg. In all the areas where the simple goiter is prevalent, there exist low iodine contents in the water, soil and food. Endemic areas in this context are Himalayan ranges in India. Besides the mountain ranges, the people living in low areas of our country are also prone to this disease because of the fact that their soils do not have enough of iodine and the water for the inhabitants comes from the mountains nearby. The plains of Manipur, Assam and other areas situated near mountains on low land are the examples. It can also be noted that calcium is also goitrogenic and goiter is common in low iodine areas where limestone or chalk is present in the soil. An interesting note is that no one can say with positive authority that the iodine deficiency is the main cause of simple goiter. It has another picture still people are having goiter in the areas where iodine is adequate in food, soil and water. The reason can be failure of intestinal absorption of iodine here. Non-absorption of iodine means deficiency of iodine in the body. This can be true in any region of the country.

PATHOLOGY

There is a great variation in the pathology depending upon different individuals at different stages of the disease and different places. There is hyperplasia of most of the normal tissues, increase in the glandular tissue, and a fibrous condition in which the interstitial tissue increases out of all proportion to other tissues, a sclerosis in very old cases, and a cystic degeneration. The cyst may be amyloidal, calcareous or colloid and fluids may be of various consistencies.

SYMPTOMS

The very first symptom of the disease is enlargement of the gland. The patient comes to the doctor to see that the disfigurement of the gland is removed. There is a fear in his or her mind that some goiters turn enormously large obstructing even the movement of the head. As written under the introduction, some goiters appear uniform in swelling but some are greater in size to the left or to the right side. There is a strange trait of the disease that the appearance of goiters is more in women and it is observed that the size of the swelling increases with each menstrual period and decreases midway between the periods. Some goiters increase during gestation and some decrease in size. The swelling or the tumor is free and mobile. They move during the act of swallowing food or water. The tumor is not adhering to the skin of the neck, the bones or the tissues of the skin. On touching there is no sensation of pain. In case the tumor is more enlarged inside the skin or the growth is small and firm but the growth inwards is more, there is sensation of discomfort due to pressure on the trachea, esophagus or upon nerves and blood vessels. The veins of the growth are large and prominent. A continuous type of headache and insomnia also feature. Till the time, inflammation, suppuration and degeneration takes place, the patient seldom feels any effects of malnutrition or ill health. The pulse rate of the patient is lower than normal and the menstrual function is abnormal. Too frequent and too profuse menses are also the symptoms of the disease along with ovaralgia, ovaritis and leucorrheal vaginitis. In some cases, frequent bouts of constipation or diarrhea are also reported.

Disorders of enzyme deficiency and synthesis of thyroid hormones

Simple goiter is also due to the defect in synthesis of thyroid hormones in which two factors play part. The first one is *enzyme deficiency* within thyroid gland and the second one is *goitrogens*.

Let us have a look at enzyme deficiency. T3 and T4 hormones are bound to thyroglobulin within the colloid and several enzymes in several steps control synthesis within the thyroglobulin complex. First the inorganic iodide is trapped from blood. The next is oxidation of iodine to iodide and binding of iodine with tyrosine to form iodotyrosines. The third step is joining of mono and di-iodotyrosines to manufacture T3 and T4. As and when the hormones are needed, thyroglobulin is broken down and the two hormones T3 and T4 are liberated to enter the blood. Here they are bound to serum proteins. A small amount of hormone remains free in serum at par with protein bound hormone. This small amount is biologically active.

Besides this, it is also possible that a family history is responsible for a simple goiter, which may be a genetic defect. On the other hand, if we remain with the theory of enzymes deficiency, it can be easily said that if iodine intake is very high in the non-endemic areas, the enzyme deficiency is overcome. Enzyme deficiency is often associated with a low iodine intake.

On the second reason given above, goitrogens are supposed to be the vegetables of the brassica family (cabbage for example), which contain thiocyanate. Taking large quantities of iodides are thought to be goitrogenic because they inhibit the organic binding of iodine and result in iodide goitre.

In the definition of simple goiter, we have classified simple goiter into two clinical types, *diffuse hyperplastic goiter* and *nodular goiter*.

TOXIC GOITER

Toxic goiter or thyrotoxicosis is basically enlargement of thyroid gland along with excessive secretion of thyroid hormones (thyroxine). The epithelial cells under the condition of disease are hypertrophied and hyperplastic. A toxic goiter may be a diffuse one, a toxic nodular goiter, or a toxic nodule. It is also called endemic goiter. Grave's disease is always associated with toxic goiter.

CLINICAL FEATURES OF TOXIC GOITER (THYROTOXICOSIS)
- Fear, anxiety and restlessness.
- One of the manifestations is tremor. When the patient holds his index finger out closing the other fingers or separating the other fingers, a tremor can be seen.
- Weight loss.

- Both heart rate and pulse rate are increased and persists during sleep, thus making it different from tachycardia. This is an important sign.
- Younger patients get this persistent tachycardia accentuated by exercise and emotions.

Ocular signs

Ocular signs are associate often although they may appear independently without thyroid overactivity. Such a condition is called *exophthalmos*. There is widening of palpebral fissure and upper eyelid partly covers the upper margin of the cornea. In usual staring, the full cornea is not exposed whereas in the case, whole of the cornea is exposed because of retraction of the upper eyelids. This makes the eyeball protrude. In some cases, edema of eyeball with congestion of eye is seen. Also in some cases, there is loss of furrows of the forehead.

Metabolism

There is increased appetite due to increased basal metabolic rate but the weight goes on reducing. Negative nitrogen balance adds to the wasting of body weight but there is no demineralization of the bones.

Gastrointestinal Manifestations

Diarrhoea of an unknown origin with discomfort in the abdomen does occur. Epigastric pain simulating gastric ulcer may also occur.

Sexual function

In males, cases of impotency are reported. In women, oligomenorrhea and amenorrhea occur in about 50 percent of cases when there is severe degree of thyrotoxicosis. Menorrhagia is rare.

DIAGNOSIS (THYROTOXICOSIS)

Check the pulse of the patient while he or she is sleeping. It will be above 90 per minute in the absence of other causes.

Normal PBI is about 3.5 to 8 g per 100 ml. An excess over 8 g is found in most of the patients. If the patient has been taking Entrovioform or Dependal tablets or other iodine containing drugs for long period, this will affect PBI.

Diffuse hyperplastic goiter is the one, which has history of endemic areas. It is soft, diffuse and generally large. In sporadic cases, it is generally found during puberty period when the metabolic demands of the body are high. Young girls and boys have this type of goiter in goiter-prone areas. From a side profile of the person, the doctor can see the hump at the neck below chin. Sometimes this type of puberty goiter goes into regression stage but appears during the period of stress in the later age, especially in girls, when pregnancy-stress becomes a cause. In this case, the TSH stimulation is less. If the TSH stimulation has totally fallen off, the diffuse goiter turns into colloid goiter. One can say that *colloid goiter* is a late stage of diffuse hyperplasia when many follicles are inactive and full of colloid due to non-stimulation of TSH.

Nodular goiter is the nodular state of goiter. We have discussed about less of stimulation and absence of stimulation of TSH resulting in diffuse and colloid states. In nodular goiter, it is again the stimulation factor of TSH wherein there is continuous or persistent fluctuation in TSH stimulation. Nodules are solitary and multiple. Most of the times they are multiple although by naked eye, they appear to be a single nodule. Under microscope, one can see the multiplication. About 50 percent are seen as multiple nodules. Ten percent are true singular. The nodules may be cellular or colloid or cystic. Degeneration of nodules and even hemorrhage is common and so is subsequent calcification. *Females are more prone to nodular goiters than men.*

The diagnosis of nodular goiter is that the nodules are palpable and often visible. They are simple, smooth, not very hard, painless, and move up and down freely when swallowing. If there is hardness and pain accompanied by features like sudden appearance, rapid enlargement of the nodule, irregular size, the suspicion of cancer does occur but most of the times such conditions are due to hemorrhage into a simple goiter. Cancer incidents are very less, say 5 to 8 percent of the cases, that too in endemic areas.

To find out the possibility of mild hyperthyroidism, the thyroid functions test should be taken up along with a straight X-ray to check tracheal compression or deviation and also calcification.

Prevention of this simple goiter in endemic areas is being looked after by respective state governments by keeping thorough check in the salt being sold there. The salt is directed to be iodized (a part of potassium iodide to be mixed in ten thousand parts of salt). The first stage of simple goiter is controllable by continued intake of medicines in allopathy but the nodular stage of simple goiter is mostly irreversible. A subtotal thyroidectomy is taken up if the patient has no multiple diseases.

OPTION FOR SURGERY

In case the goiter is large, the thyroid is overactive and under such condition, goiter is pressing the windpipe. If the goiter is of medium size but is a cause of uneasiness or the intake of drugs have been bothering you since the relief is not in sight, it is better to go in for surgery, of course, on the advice of doctor, this advise will be forthcoming if you happen to plan for a baby birth. A partial thyroidectomy is supposed to be an effective treatment for hyperthyroidism and protruding goiter.

In partial thyroidectomy, about two third of each of the two lobes of the thyroid are removed. Before the surgery, the doctor ensures that thyroid levels are normal. It is done by means of induction of antithyroid drugs and iodine compound (a solution of iodine and potassium iodine in water). The vocal cord is also checked before the examination. Most of the doctors detach the glands from the blood supply and remove more rather than less of the thyroid to avoid recurring episodes of overactivity and need for subsequent surgery. In many cases, thyroidectomy restores normal thyroid function. The overall health condition is also seen in such cases and mostly young women having this problem are advised to go in for surgery. Not all surgeries yield fruitful results. It depends upon the skill of the surgeon and his experience. Two to five percent of the surgery cases face a failure. About five in hundred patients may experience recurrent episodes of overactivity from time to time. In surgery, utmost care is taken that while operating upon thyroid, there is no harm caused deep into parathyroid glands. It is these glands, which control calcium balance in the body. If these glands are disturbed, there can be an acute worse condition. Besides this, there is some risk of damage to the nerves and vessels which supply blood to vocal cords. If the operation is in skilled hands, such complications do not occur.

HOMEOPATHIC TREATMENT FOR GOITER

The main remedies for goiter are *Iodium, Spongia tosta, Fluoricum acidum, Calcarea iodatum, Calcarea carbonica, Bromium, Kalium iodatum* and *Calcarea fluorica* and *Fucus vesiculosa*.

The main remedies for exophthalmus are *Amylenum nitrosum, Belladonna, Dubois, Ferrum phosphoricum, Lycopus virginicus,* and *Natrium muriaticum.*

Iodium

Iodium acts mainly on the glandular and lymphatic system, stimulating them at first to an increased action, which is soon followed by marked depression, emaciation and atrophy, There is ravenous appetite with great emaciation and it acts on the gland causing enlargement. It is quite useful in goiter. *(W.A. Dewey in*

Essentials of Homoeopathic Materia Medica and Homoeopathic Pharmacy—B Jain publishers).

Hypertrophy runs through the remedy. There is enlargement of the liver, spleen, ovaries, testes, lymphatic glands, and cervical glands, of all the glands except the mammary glands. The mammae dwindle while all other glands become enlarged, nodular and hard. The enlargement of the glands is especially observed among the lymphatic glands of the abdomen, the mesenteric glands. There is this peculiar circumstance also in Iodium, viz., "that while the body withers the glands enlarge." This is a description made by Kent in his book 'Lectures on Homoeopathic Materia Medica.'

Geroge Royal in his book 'Homoeopathic Theory and Practice of Medicine,' recommends Iodine for goiters in the following fashion:

The Iodium patient has dark hair, yellow, tawny skin, is spare, as a rule emaciated. The glands or glandular organs especially affected are the mesentery, the pancreas, and the liver. Iodium produces a tendency to atrophy with induration, while *Bromium* has enlargement with softening. Instead of producing large, soft tumors in the mammary glands, it produces small hard tumors or nodes in the skin of those glands. The Iodium patients are depressed, low-spirited, suicidal, while the *Bromium* patient is more buoyant, and cheerful. She may have all sorts of delusions but of things outside herself. Do not give Iodium too low, the 12th is low enough, the 30th is better in most cases. Three times daily is enough.

Boericke's Materia Medica identifies the remedy as one of the best for goiters.

Rapid metabolism, loss of flesh with great appetite. Hungry with much thirst. Better after eating. Great debility, the slightest effort induces perspiration. Iodium individual is exceedingly thin, dark complexioned, with enlarged lymphatic glands, has voracious appetite but gets thin. Tubercular type. It has acute exacerbation of chronic inflammation. Acts prominently on connective tissue, the plague and goiters. Larynx feels constricted. Eustachian deafness. Thyroid enlarged. Goiter with sensation of constriction. Swollen submaxillary glands and uvula swollen.

Whenever this remedy is indicated, one can notice the marked emaciation and ravenous hunger, a type which cannot be satisfied. Protrusion of the eyeballs with violent palpitation of the heart, worse on exertion and a constant, heavy, oppressive pain in the region of the heart. The pulse is rapid, small, weak and often irregular. All diseases demanding this remedy are characterized by *torpidity*.

Iodium is very valuable remedy in goiters and especially so in the beginning or when the tumor is soft. It is also of value later on. Many cures have been made with infinitesimal doses of this remedy and many a mineral spring has made its reputation for cure of goiters from minute amount of iodine that is contained. (Plain talks on Materia Medica with comparison by *Willard Ide Pierce* – B. Jain Publishers)

Hering says on Iodium, *"Inveterate cases of goiter, the harder they feel and the more other symptoms are wanting, the better indicated."*

Allen H.C. warns that local application of iodine to the goiter is not desired. While the size of the tumor is reduced by local application, there have followed alarming pulmonary symptoms. Allen also recommends this remedy for *hard goiter in black haired person* (in light haired persons, it is *Bromium*).

E.B. Nash in his book 'Leaders in homoeopathic therapeutics' gives an assurance that *Iodium* is the best remedy. He says, "It makes no difference whether it is phthisis pulmonalis, mesenteric, or general, but this symptom well developed rules out everything but *Iodium* in almost every case and it has made many remarkable cures. *I have cured many cases of goiter with Iodium C.M., when* indicated, giving a powder every night for four nights, after the moon fulled and was waning. I have failed in one case either to check the further development or cure. Some will sneer at this, but the cured ones do not. The local application for glandular enlargement is foolish and dangerous."

Lippe says that *Iodium* acts best in goiter when given after full moon, or when the moon is waning. It may be noted that Nash also recommends the same.

Rai Bahadur Bishamber Das in his book, 'Select your remedy' has a remarkable description of *Iodium*. Please note that he recommends 1 M potency, "*Iodium* is the head remedy for goiter and is indicated in spare dark, active patients. *It should be given in 1 M dilution.* Marked hardness with sensation of constriction. Hypertrophy of two lobes, tumor becoming more swollen and painful at each return of menses. Glandular increase in size, especially the right side, soft and without any fluctuation. Non-lobulated tumor in interior and medium portion of the size as large as a child's head, rosy red, heavy in weight and soft is cured by this remedy. Patient is thin but eats heartily. Goiter soft with heat and rapid pulse. The Iodium patients are depressed, low spirited and suicidal.

N.C. Ghosh in 'Comparative Materia Medica' gives an important indication of use of *Iodium* in goiters. The swelling is big in size, hard to touch and there is no pain.

K.C. Bhanja in his 'Homoeopathic Prescriber' states that *Iodium* patient cannot remain seated or at times even sleep.

J.N. Shinghal in his book 'Bedside Prescriber' considers *Iodium* as a classical remedy for goiter.

Iodium is a classical remedy for goiter, simple and exophthalmic variety, which include thyroid enlargement, tachycardia and tremors. It is useful in simple soft variety of goiter and here it should be used low and in the indurated varieties, better results are seen with the use of higher potency. The external use of iodine is harmful. As per homoeopathic view of most of scholars, Goiter and Grave's disease are not surgical diseases.

Spongia tosta

A long-term used remedy by many homoeopaths in the treatment of enlarged thyroid is *Spongia*. In the past, especially in America, the villagers used to take *Spongia*. It contains iodine. In the valleys where goiter abounded, people were using a powder containing powdered egg-shell (*Calcarea carbonica*), burnt sponge (*Spongia tosta*) and sugar. This type of treatment has many successful results on record.

Why *Spongia* goes in favor of goiters? It is mostly known as a heart remedy, a remedy for respiratory disorders and hypertrophy. In fact, *Spongia* has cardiac tremors as its characteristic, which is also the similar symptom in Grave's disease.

Kent has given a description of *Spong.* as follows:

'*Spongia* patient is worse in a warm room and from heat. The patient wants to be cool like *Iodium* but is better from warm drinks (*Ars., Nux-v., Lyc.*)

Spongia has a tendency to affect the glands in a striking way. Glands which are gradually increasing in size and become stony or undergo hypertrophy. *Spongia* is more suitable for patients with inflammatory diseases of the heart resulting in rheumatism in case they develop goiter. Hypertrophy of the thyroid, goiter, when the heart is affected and the eyes are protruding.

George Royal says, "Let us consider it for comparison with *Bromine*. While *Spongia* has a striking individuality, combining the characteristics of both. *Bromium* and *Iodium* makes it up. It has the complexion and glandular enlargement of *Bromium* but the mental anxiety and low vitality of *Iodium*. The action upon the respiratory organs is nearly the same for all the three.

Amenorrhea with asthmatic difficulties is found in *Spongia* rather than menorrhagia. The 2nd or 3rd is the best potency."

"Thyroid gland is swollen and hard, with suffocative attacks at night. Stitching pains and pressure. Goiter causes asthma. Pain on swallowing." Tells Dr. Balaram Jana.

Boericke states that thyroid gland is swollen. There are stitches and dryness with burning and stinging. Sore throat, worse after eating sweet things. Tickling causes cough. Clears the throat constantly.

Allen H.C. recommends *Spongia* for goiters and swollen thyroid gland even with chin; with suffocative paroxysm at night.

R.B. Bishambar Das states usefulness of *Spongia* when the goiter is painful. Pain on swallowing and the patients are inhabitants of valleys. It has the complexion and glandular enlargement of *Bromium* and the mental anxiety and low vitality of *Iodium*.

E.B. Nash says that *Spongia* is also a good remedy for goiter with sense of suffocation after sleep.

N.C. Ghosh calls *Spongia* as not a wasteful medicine, which to some experts, cures goiter in two or three doses. When thyroid gland is affected along with tumor on the neck, *Spongia* is useful.

Bhanja K.C. recommends *Spongia* when thyroid gland is swollen and hard with suffocative attacks at night. Stiching pains and pressure is also felt. Goiter causes asthma in some cases and there is pain on swallowing.

J.N. Singhal considers this remedy when the goiter is painful with pain on swallowing. The patients should be given a dose of *Spongia* at night and in the morning for a week then pause for a week and then repeat.

Fucus vesiculosus

Fucus vesiculosus is said to be 'stock' remedy for goiter whereas for exophthalmos, the remedy is *Lycopus virginicus* (Royal). *Boericke* considers this remedy both for non-toxic goiter and exophthalmic goiter. The remedy is considered for *thyroid enlargement in obese subjects*. Now compare it with *Spong.* which has iodine as its chief ingredient. *Fucus* has other ingredients, which have changed the makeup of the remedy completely. *Iodium* patient is mostly dark, active and spare, *Fucus* patient is obese, flabby and lazy. Next to the enlarged gland, disturbances of digestion are most common and these are constipation and flatulence. The constipation is quite obstinate and forehead feels as if compressed by an iron ring. It is important that the dose be taken in five to sixty drops of the tincture a few minutes before meals and three times a day. Many doctors prefer to use *Bromium, Iodium* and *Spongia* instead of *Fucus* because of the fact that the patient does not present subjective symptoms.

Bromium

Bromium is although a chief remedy for respiratory symptoms with affection of larynx and trachea yet its importance cannot be ignored in scrofulous children with enlarged parotid and goiter *(Boericke)*.

Geroge Royal says that the Bromide patient is light complexioned, large, and scrofulous. In addition to the thyroid gland, there is usually a history of troubles with the parotid, the mammary, the ovary, the testicles and the tonsils in the order named. The enlargement of the parotid, the tumors in the breasts, as well as the thyroid gland, are all aggravated by the menses, which are too early and too profuse, also worse from warm weather and better in open sea air. It works better in 3rd potency and makes a fresh preparation each time for each patient. *There is also a caution that milk should not be given to the Bromium patient.*

E.B. Nash does not recommend this remedy for goiter but states that it is good for glandular affections as are Carbo animalis and Conium. Both these and Bromium are for stony hard glands with cancerous tendency.

Bhanja says that *Bromium* should be considered for *goiter of the size of hen's egg*. The swelling is very hard. For stony hardness of the goiter, he also recommends *Calcarea fluorica*.

According to R.B. Bishambar Das, when *Iodium* in 1 M dilution fails, this remedy, *Bromium* should be tried in high dilutions viz., 1 M. There is enlargement of the glands with softness, one cannot lie on the right side because of palpitations and the patient is light complexioned, scrofulous, buoyant and cheerful.

It is worth nothing here that while Nash states that *Bromium* is indicated in stony hard glands, Das says the opposite i.e. softness of gland. The reason appears to be that Nash does not recommend it for goiter but general glands or tumors.

Calcarea carbonica

In simple goiter, in those of strumous diathesis, this remedy has been used successfully. Cured cases on record are numerous according to Dr. Zopfy of Germany.

Boericke considers this great anti-psoric constitutional remedy *par excellence*, if the symptoms and constitution agree with the patient of goiter, thyroid and pituitary dysfunction.

George Royal states that it is a leading remedy for that strumous, scrofulous goiter patients who are deficient in lime salts. The patient is even more flabby and fat than the *Spongia* patient. Not only the thyroid but also the other glands are larger and softer than normal. Similar is the condition of muscles and bones. With the glandular system, the skin and the organs of digestion suffer, and acidity is the most pronounced result. Sour eructation, sour vomitus, sour stools, sour sweat are all prominent symptoms of *Calcarea carbonica*. The uterine symptoms are also prominent in the goiter group. The menses are early and profuse, the leucorrhea is also profuse. The mental state is low. Fear of going crazy, forgetfulness and apprehension are the leading symptoms, together with the enlargement of the goiter are all much worse just before each menstrual period. Royal prefers 12th trituration twice daily or the 30th dilution once daily.

Bhanja K.C. says that this remedy is useful when swelling is hard and worst towards new moon in scrofulous persons.

Dr. Zopfy of Germany claims that *Calcarea carbonica* will cure most simple cases (*Bedside Prescriber by Shinghal*).

R.B. Bishamber Das says that it is useful in simple goiters in fat persons with sweating on the head and neck. *It may be given in 200 dilution every two hours six times daily until improvement starts.*

Calcarea iodatum

George Royal has this to say about *Calcarea iodatum*. Like *Spongia* it is another hybrid, a mixture of *Calc* and *Iod*, the earmarks of the latter being much more prominent than those of the former. The glands are smaller and firmer than under *Calc*area *carbonica* the bones are weak as are those of *Calc*area *carbonica* but the cause of weakness is lack of material and improper distribution of a sufficient or even an over – abundance of supply. The *Calcarea iodatum* patient is dark instead of light complexioned. The tumors of the mammary glands, which frequently accompany goiters are nodular, freely movable, very tender to touch and excruciatingly painful when moving the arm. All glandular manifestations are worse before the menses flow. He used the 3rd or 6th trituration. According to him, *Trillium*, Billing's and Clapp's oxide of lime, *Kali bi.* and *Phyt.* are the four remedies belonging to the *Calc.* class, useful for a tense firm enlargement of the thyroid.

Dr. Zopfy of Germany says that it is a useful remedy for *goiters* and it should be given one dose a week. Then there should be a wait to see the result before repeating it weekly.

Ferrum iodatum

According to Boericke, scrofulous affections, glandular enlargement and tumors call for this remedy. Crops of boils, acute nephritis following eruptive diseases, uterine displacement and exophthalmic goiter following suppression of menses are some of the symptoms for this remedy.

According to *Kent*, the remedy is useful in exophthalmic goiter provided the other symptoms agree. The symptoms like burning, pressing, tickling and scraping in the throat with swollen cervical glands are indicative of the remedy.

Ferr-i. is indicated when there is disturbance in the female sexual organs and when the menses are scanty or suppressed. The body is emaciated and anemia is also present. Many a times it has cured exophthalmic goiter following suppression of the menses. (*Dr. Balaram Jana in Essential of Practice of Medicines –B. Jain Publishers*)

Rai Bahadur Bishamber Das does not find *Ferr-i.* useful for exophthalmic goiter but on the other hand he recommends *Ferr.* useful especially after suppression of menses.

Lycopus virginicus

Many homoeopaths recommend this remedy in a high tone for treatment of exophthalmic variety of goiter. Its main indications or symptoms are constriction of chest, weak pulse, which is remittent, tremulous and rapid. Sometimes, the heart's action is tumultous and forcible. *Jousset*, a known homoeopath of America esteems it highly for well-marked cases of exophthalmos.

Boericke says that this remedy lowers the blood pressure, reduces the rate of heart and increases the length of systole to a great degree. It is a heart remedy but of use in exophthalmic goiter.

Dr. Balaram Jana says that this remedy is probably indicated more frequently than any other. When there is rapid pulse, abnormal cardiac action, heart being tumultous and forcible. There is cough and often hemoptysis. It gives the best results when given in five-drop doses of the tincture every three hours.

Lycopodium clavatum

The tumor or the swelling of goiter is on the right side. It is tense, smooth and shining with a feeling of constriction. The swelling is not very large. (*Bishambar Das*)

"Abnormal protrusion of eye balls, sensitive to heat, desires hot food, aggravation of symptoms in warm room, diarrhea after heavy meals, menses irregular or profuse and painful and liking for sweets are some of the symptoms when accompanying goiter (exophthalmic)", says *J.N. Shinghal.*

Natrium muriaticum

In patients who have palpitation of the heart and the heart-beat seems to shake the entire body. This salt is useful in exophthalmic goiter in subjects of a cachectic appearance. Natrium mur. is likely to be useful remedy to finish and fix the cure begun by some other remedy.

The peculiar symptoms in early stages of goiter is that the patient is afraid of thunderstorm. He or she is also afraid to be alone at night. His or her heart rate slows down when using stethoscope and accelerates when the pulse rate is counted. Exophthalmic goiter with emaciation, weakness, trembling, palpitation, thirst, nervous irritability and sleeplessness are its symptoms. (*Bishambar Das*)

Adrenalinum

Bishamber Das is sure of its usefulness in exophthalmic goiter wherein there is quick pulse, rapid heart action and dyspnea. Eyeballs are protruding and there is throbbing of the arteries at the back of the neck. *Adren.* may be given in 200 or 1M dilution. If this fails try *Cact.*

Thyroidinum

Thyroidinum has plenty of anemia, emaciation, sweating and persistent frontal headache and muscular weakness. This remedy brings forth a regulatory influence over nutrition, growth and development. Basedow tachycardia and exophthalmic goiter with palpitation from the least excitement, easy excitability of the heart and dry skin are the symptoms of this remedy. It is a belief that high potencies are more efficient in the exophthalmic variety and much safer than the taking of the crude thyroid which has a large element of danger. This remedy also reinforces the action of *Lycopus virginicus* and is complemented by *Fucus vesiculosus.*

According to *Bishamber Das*, this remedy may be tried when *Iod.* and *Brom.* fail. Give 3x or 6x trituration.

Thyr. is useful in goiter cases where obesity is present and the patient is pale. *(Boericke)*

The remedy is suitable for fat, debilitated and anemic persons, who suffers from weakness and palpitation from least exertion. Two or three doses of *Thyr.* 3x should be given per day for some days and it is to be repeated after some gap watching the pulse rate. This remedy reinforces the action of *Lycps.*, and is complemented by *Fuc.* (*J.N. Singhal*)

Lapis albus

This remedy corresponds to simple goiter of a soft doughy (flour kneaded with water) feel, rather than the hard indurated encapsulated varieties.

Lapis albus is silico fluoride of calcium and was first recommended by *Grauvogl* for treatment of goiter as it formed an important constituent of water of Swiss valley where goiter w prevalent. *Hale* later recommended the remedy. This remedy is also useful in certain forms of enlarged glands about the throat. Anemia is an indication for its use and it acts best in 6th trituration. It is of less use for stony hard goiter. (*W.A. Dewey – Essentials of Homoeopathic Materia Medica and Homoeopathic Pharmacy, B. Jain*)

Goiter in which burning is reported and stinging pain is expressed in breasts, stomach and uterus. Scrofulous enlargement of glands. (*Bishamber Das*)

Boericke calls for this remedy in the case of affections of glands, goiter, and other connected diseases. Goiter has a certain elasticity and pliability about them rather than stony hardness of *Calc-f.* and *Con.*

Lap-a. increases markedly the appetite and suits well persons of anemic tendency.

Ignatia amara

When there is pain in goiter in nervous patients, *Ign.* may be tried. (*Bishamber Das*)

Also check the other symptoms of *Ign.*

BIOCHEMIC AND HOMOEOPATHIC COMBINATIONS FOR GOITER

B.S. Darbari in his book 'Simple remedies' has given a useful combination of biochemic remedies. Mixture of Calc-f 3x, Calc-p 3x, Mag-p 3x, Nat-m 3x and Sil. 12x should be given for two weeks. If it does no good for two weeks, 1 pill of *Iod.* 200 on the day next to full moon; and repeat it again next day after next full moon; and so on 3 or 4 doses; if this fails give *Iod.* 1000 – 1 pill to be given in the similar manner.

VIEWS OF GEORGE ROYAL

George Royal in his book, 'Homoeopathic Theory and Practice of medicine' has given a summary of the disease and its treatment in an established manner. This is a short summary.

"Enlargement of the gland is the first symptom noticed and the patient seeks the physician to prevent disfigurement rather than because of any subjective manifestation, because the patient knows that some goiters attain enormous size, sometimes hanging over the chest and in other ways hindering the motion of the head. The enlargement may be uniform or greater on the right side or in the middle. The size may vary at intervals. The great majority, which have come under my care increase with each menstrual period and decrease midway between the periods; some increase during gestation and some decrease. As a rule, the tumor is free and movable, which may be determined by directing the patient to conduct the act of swallowing. It does not adhere to the skin; bones or other tissues till after some degenerative process have taken place. Handling the gland causes no pain. The sensation of discomfort, due to pressure on the trachea, esophagus or upon the nerves and blood vessels, are more pronounced in those patients when the growth is small and firm but growing inward than when the tumor is large, soft and growing outward from the gland. The veins of the growth are larger and prominent. The patient seldom feels any effects of malnutrition or ill health until inflammation, suppuration and degeneration takes place or until some needless and improper operation has been performed, when many of the symptoms of myxedema and sepsis may appear. These symptoms may be simple insomnia, severe, continuous headache, or marked brain and nervous symptoms like convulsions or tetany, the latter the result of injudicious treatment. The only exception being that the function of the thyroid has been destroyed by the disease and not by the knife. The pulse rate in the usual complicated cases is usually slower than the normal; in one case of mine, as low as 35, and generally full, also regular. The menstrual function is rarely normal. The most frequent variation being too frequent and too profuse menses. Ovaralgia, ovaritis, and chronic leucorrheal vaginitis are also common symptoms. In a certain proportion of cases, I would say one-third disturbances of the alimentary canal are in evidence, a tendency to acidity, to constipation or diarrhea. In a still smaller percentage of cases, we have dryness and roughness of the skin and occasionally profuse perspiration."

REPERTORY SUGGESTIONS

GOITER

Kent in his repertory has mentioned 54 remedies in general to treat goiter. It is very difficult as to find out the exact remedy in this fashion. In order to ease this situation, he has mentioned remedies preferring sides and nature of pains, etc. Here is a list of remedies in that fashion.

Goiter – Right sided: *Caust., Hep., Iod., Mag-c., Merc-i-f., Nat-c, Phos., Sep., Sil., Spong.*

Left sided: *Chel., Lach.*

Constriction: *Calc-s., Crot-c., Iod., Lys., Spong.*

Exophthalmic: *Aur., Aur-i., Cact., Calc., Con., Crot-h., Ferr., Ferr-i., Ferr-p., Iod., Lycps., Nat-m., Phos., Scut., Sec., Spong., Thyr.*

Indurated: *Iod., Spong.*

Menses before, agg.: *Cimic.*

Painful: *Iod., Plat., Spong.*

Painful, menses during: *Iod.*

Painful, swallowing on: *Spong.*

Pressing: *Nat-c.*

Pulsation: *Iod., Lyc.*

Sensitive *Kali-i.*
Tickling *Plat.*
Twitching *Lyc.*
Vascular *Apis., Calc.*

GENERAL

At the age of puberty when patient is susceptible to cold: *Calc-i*

Goiter, from suppressed menses: *Ferr-i.*

Obese and constipated persons: *Fuc. Q*

Hard with feeling as if air inhaled is passing through the goiter, pain in heart regions also with a choking feeling in the throat: *Spong.*

Painful goiter, swollen and with emaciation even though eating well, swelling and pain worse during menses, slowly increasing size: *Iod.*

Goiter, with cardiac symptoms: *Cact. Q*

Right sides with sensitiveness to all impressions and patient chilly: *Hep.*

Goiter big as the size of egg of the hen: *Brom.*

Goiter hard swollen worse during menses: *Calc.*

Goiter, nodular with swelling: *Phyt.*

Goiter, pressing pains, with swelling on upper side: *Nat-c.*

THYROIDITIS

GRANULOMATOUS THYROIDITIS

The *granulomatous thyroiditis* is due to viral infection. There is irregular enlargement of one or both thyroid lobes. Fever, pain in the neck, raised ESR and T4 is slightly raised but the overall condition is self-limiting.

Within a few months, the goiter subsides and any subsequent hypothyroidism is a rare phenomenon. In some cases, the condition of the pains are acute, the goiter is painful. In most of the cases, the pain killer tablets are given along with the antibiotic course if one resorts to allopathy.

HASHIMOTO'S THYROIDITIS

Hashimoto's disease is an auto immune disorder first described by Hashimoto. It is more common than the granulomatous thyroiditis. It is well characterized by chronic inflammation of the thyroid and goiter formation. It is mostly associated with the family history of autoimmune diseases like pernicious anemia, autoimmune gastritis and thyrotoxicosis. It is more common in women than men. As a matter of fact, it has relation with antibodies of thyroid gland. In normal persons, thyroid antibodies may be present in low levels. Low levels are not diagnostic of autoimmune disease. Autoimmune thyroiditis has raised levels of thyroid antibodies. Clinical tests like C.F.T (complement fixation test) and T.R.C. (Tanned red cell) are available for this.

Autoimmune thyroiditis can be classified into three categories (I) focal (II) Non diffuse goiter, and (III) diffuse goiter (lymphadenoid goiter or Hashimoto's disease) thyroiditis.

The **symptoms of Hashimoto's** *thyroiditis* are presence of a smooth goiter without pain and not of much large size due to which there is less of pressure felt by the patient. The surrounding skin and the structure are not much changed. With the progress of disease, the gland becomes fibrotic and impalpable and may present with myxedema. The patient is usually in normal state but initially there may be brief period of hyper-thyroidism.

Diagnosis

Hashimoto's disease is mostly confused with non-toxic goiter. The late onset of the disease and high antibody titre serve as a distinction from non-toxic goiter.

HOMOEOPATHIC TREATMENT

Homoeopathic remedies for the treatment of thyroiditis are those, which have an affinity for the thyroid and have the power to check the inflammation, to regulate the circulation, to prevent the formation of and cause the absorption of pus.

To check the inflammation, we have Aconitum napellus, Belladonna atropa, Thyroidinum, Phytolaca decandra and Ferrum phosphoricum. To prevent suppuration, we have Hepar sulphuris 30 & Silicea terra 30 or any of the remedies whose indication are given under the heading of sepsis.

Homoeopathic treatment is based upon the symptoms and the main remedy in this diseases is *Thyroidinum* 3x. It is especially indicated in people, who suffer from anemia, are depressed to the core, suffer from muscular weakness and get palpitation on least exertion. Such patients also have edematous extremities and are chilly. Thyroidinum, when inducted in such patients may increase their body weight. Once this starts, the doctor should recognize that the medicine is working. In case this medicine does not work, the medicines given in the therapeutics of *'Goiter'* in the last chapter should be tried according to the symptoms.

VIEWS OF GEORGE ROYAL ON THYROIDITIS

Thyroiditis or Strumitis (this term is used when the gland has been previously diseased but the two are used as synonym) may be an acute congestion or repeated attacks of the congestion or repeated attacks of both. Rarely, the cause is trauma, but the great majority of cases are secondary to infectious diseases like typhoid, small pox, malaria etc. Often, the infection may be the result of aspirating with a needle or using one for electricity.

The many blood vessels are engorged; also hemorrhages and thrombi, all of which make the gland swollen and boggy. The tissue then breaks down and abscesses form.

Symptoms:

At first severe pain extending to the ears, fever, marked local tenderness, swelling, headache, vertigo, epistaxis; then suppuration and pus in one or the other of the lobes. The abscess may rupture and discharge into the oesophagus or trachea. All the symptoms are more severe in strumitis than thyroiditis. Most writers give two pathognomonic symptoms of abscesses in addition to the general symptoms of suppuration, viz., "limitation of chin elevation and depression of the chin on the sternum when swallowing". We may also have many symptoms of pressure on the trachea and the esophagus due to pressure of the enlarged gland; cyanosis is common.

Diagnosis

Simple congestion and laryngeal perichondritis may be mistaken for this disease. The former is caused by the interference of the circulation with tight collars or bands, or by emotional and menstrual disturbances and may thus be readily recognized and excluded.

Prognosis

It is favourable as a rule. The exception are those cases in which the pus is discharged into the trachea or esophagus. In rare instances, myxedema may result when the gland has been destroyed by the disease or entirely removed in an operation.

The homoeopathic remedies suggest by *George Royal*, mentioned previously, are in the auxiliary treatment. His views are quite beneficial. He says that extreme heat or cold should be applied to the first stage. Tincture of *Arnica* may also be used both locally and internally. When used locally, the solution is one part of the tincture to four parts of water and should be used as hot as possible. Other treatment consists in the evacuation of pus and the removal of the part of the gland. Tracheotomy may be required.

Hypothyroidism Myxedema

HYPO MEANING deficiency and thyroid the gland; in other words, it is *lack of thyroid hormones caused by an under-active thyroid gland.* The term *myxedema* is a condition of hypothyrodism occurring in middle-aged individuals, usually females. It may occur endemically or sporadically. There are two types of hypothyroidism, *primary and secondary.*

The *primary* is due to malfunction of thyroid proper and *the secondary* is malfunction of the gland due to defects in hypothalamus and/or pituitary glands. We shall discuss about primary hypothyroidism at present *(Secondary hypothyroidism is discussed on page* 89). Hypothyroidism favours women than men. The conditions leading to this disease are such that patient does not know that she/he is suffering from this disease and make a wrong estimate to general debility, tiredness and overwork or tension. The symptoms it produces are mostly confusing and the first symptom that strikes is depression. One feels as his or her mental energy has gone down and that he or she needs a change from her domestic or office work. From day to day, the energy level of the person fluctuates. *If you want to term this disease in better diagnostic feature, it can be said that all systems get slow in this disease and that too softly, that you would not know what is happening to the body.*

DISORDERS OF HYPOTHYROIDISM

There are three major disorders in hypothyroidism:
- Myxedema*
- Myxedema in childhood
- Cretinism**

*The term **Myxedema** is explained in the following headings under differential diagnosis. However, in short we can say that signs and symptoms of hypothyroidism are accentuated (stress of the voice). There is a typical facial appearance showing clavicular puffiness, a sort of malar flush (pertaining to cheeks) and a yellow tinge to the skin. The body temperature goes down and the patient has to be warmed up slowly in cold climates and cold countries.

Cretinism in literal meaning is dwarfishness. Cretinism is a classification of hypothyroidism. It may be infantile or fetal. There may be total or near total absence of the growth of the thyroid development and in such cases, the possibility is that the parents and their other children may have normal growth and functioning of thyroid. In endemic areas Goitrous cretinism is due to maternal reasons and fetal iodine deficiency. Such cases have peculiar state of body appearance when born. Infantile cretinism children have pale, puffy face, pot-bellied with umbilical hernia seen prominently. Their tongue remains protruded and lips have a swollen appearance. Certain subject in the adulthood is mentally and physically retarded. They have pads of fats as if layers of skin upon skin in the clavicular areas. The skin is dry and wrinkled.

ETIOLOGY

Complete removal of the thyroid gland leads to the condition called hypothyroidism. A partial removal of the gland also amount to it but the remainder of the gland atrophies although the cause of atrophy is not known. It is also seen that if one member is found to be suffering from hypothyroidism, there is likelihood of other members of the family having the same disease at a different stage, matured or in the stage of maturity while not knowing the exact symptoms. Hypothyroidism is mostly the disease associated with cold climate and in countries having cool and temperate zones than in warm countries. This fact has its own doubts. The slower metabolism, the main cause of this disease, cannot be fully attributed to cold climate, rather its jaws are spreading to warm countries. The reason why more cases of hypo or hyperthyroidsm are designated can be attributed to quick diagnostic measures in developed countries. In hot countries and in the Asian region, the thyroid disease is not quickly diagnosed due to ignorance about the disease on the part of the patient rather than the doctor. Females are more affected than the males and according to an old estimate in America, the ratio of women to men is 7:1 and the common age for both the sexes is 35 to 50 years. In young children, the atrophy is observed in thyroid, which can stimulate cretinism. In another survey conducted by the British general practitioners, 9 out of 1000 women suffer from the conditions called hypothyroidism. On the other hand, only one out of thousand men suffer from this disease. Accurate figures in India are not known because of diagnostic difficulties (owing to patient's own lethargy), but according to an estimate 25 out of 1000 women suffers from this disease. For men, the figures are not available. In another estimate, the disease occurs in the *middle age*, being *4 to 7 times commoner in females.*

It is not fully known as to how the body turns against itself and produces this disease. Why the thyroid wastes away and shrinks and why women are more prone to this disease is still a mystery. Is it due to autoantibodies or effects of autoimmune process that body turns against its own tissues, as if they were foreign? The defense system of the body is very complicated. There are some types of white blood cells (lymphocytes), which produce immunity, or we can say that they produce resistance against the disease. Each of the cell of the body has a sort of recognition according to which the white blood cells treat them as 'self' and leave them alone. When a virus of bacteria attacks the body, the immune system recognizes them and declares them as foreign. It is then the function of lymphocytes (T) is to destroy the infections. The lymphocytes have been designed to recognize and distinguish the body's own tissues from the invaders. Due to some reason, if such quality of distincution between a friend and foe is lost, the result is a disease. Cancer is the best example of such an invasion. However, the system of homoeopathy differs from all these theories and considers every infection due to weaker vital force. This we shall take up when the treatment under homoeopathy comes up.

In a nutshell, there are four main reasons, which could give rise to hypothyrodism.

1. Hashimoto's disease*.
2. Partial or total thyroidectomy.
3. Idiopathic thyroid fibrosis.
4. Prolonged iodine therapy.

*The definition of Hashimoto is already discussed in the previous chapter dealing with goiter. However, a brief summary here will make the readers update for its connection with hypothyroidism. Hashimoto's disease is a common condition in adults with which hypothyroidism occurs. This condition in which the inflammation of the thyroid occurs is sometimes called Hashimoto's thyroiditis and it is more common in females. Women become its victim five or six times more than the men. When the inflammation occurs, there may not be initial uncomfortable feeling but there exists development of a small goiter on the neck. As the goiter increases and becomes tender, one feels uncomfortable and finds swallowing difficult. The symptoms in Hashimoto's disease have symptoms of an overactive thyroid. These symptoms will be discussed in hyperthyrodism. Hashimoto's disease has already been discussed shortly under the heading thyroiditis.

CLASSIFICATION OF HYPOTHYROIDISM

ENDEMIC CRETINISM

This is often goitrous.

FAILURE OF THYROID DEVELOPMENT

It may be complete or may be partial.

AUTOIMMUNE THYROIDITIS

It is both non-goitrous and goitrous. It is also called primary or atropathic myxedema. It is autoimmune disease like lymphadenoid goiter but without goiter formation from TSH stimulation. There is a delay in diagnosis of this state and hence hypothyroidism is much more severe than the goitrous autoimmune thyroid.

IATROGENIC

It occurs either after radioiodine therapy, pituitary ablation, thyroidectomy or induction of drugs.

VASCULAR DAMAGE TO ANTERIOR PITUITARY

Such damages may be genetic.

DYSHORMONOGENESIS AND GOITROGENS

These are deficiencies in the enzymes controlling the synthesis of thyroid hormones and mostly genetically determined. In severe conditions, they result in goiter formation and finally into hypothyroidism. If the state is mild and not severe, a simple goiter results. Such simple goiters may be with or without hypothyroidism.

EFFECTS OF DRUGS

Besides the above causes, there are other factors resulting in hypothyroidism. They are due to some *drugs* (iodine compounds, carbimazole, or lithium etc.), *cancer of thyroid, and congential* causes, which include absence of thyroid, metabolic defect and abnormal development of thyroid. *Pituitary and hypothalamic problem*s are the secondary causes.

CHILDBIRTH AND PREGNANCY

During pregnancy or after the birth of the child, the thyroid has a tendency to slow down its functioning. This same slow functioning can also occur after abortion. The problems related to hypothyroidism are rare during pregnancy. If the functioning of thyroid is slow, even conceiving is difficult. The common condition is autoimmune disease, Hashimoto's disease or if the patient had some thyroid surgery for an overactive thyroid. It is the nature of the body to improve the conditions laid by Hashimoto disease and the thyroid works quite efficiently during pregnancy. With the advance of medical science, today the conditions are different and there is a better management of both thyroid problems and complications in pregnancy.

During pregnancy, a woman requires extra thyroid hormone and may develop hypothyroidism. A women already having hypothyroidism can worsen during pregnancy.

HYPOTHYROIDISM BY BIRTH (CONGENITAL)

Congenital cases of hypothyroidism are very rare, say about one in seven thousand (figures from American survey), still the congenital causes cannot be ruled out. Such babies are born with an under-active thyroid or suffer from *thyroiditis* (inflammation of the thyroid), which may be development in the womb. After birth, the inflammation does not improve fully. There is certainly a hormonal or genetic connection to this sort of problem in newborn babies. The day is not far when advancement of *medical science equipped with gene therapy* will be able to handle this type of congenital disease. Earlier this sort of problem in babies used to be categorized as cretins but now this is not termed likewise and thyroiditis is the word used. This runs in the families but there are exceptions too. Some new-born babies have endemic goiter on account of synthesis of hormones, which is a sure sign of disorder relating to metabolism.

CANCER OF THYROID

The name cancer itself is cruel and a matter of terror for

anyone but one must bear in mind that cancer of thyroid is very rare. It tends to remain localized and does not spread. A surgeon can remove it and there are high chances of cure. In some cases, cancer is controlled with thyroid pills to put a stop to its growth and decrease the size of infection. Negligible cases are reported in instances where throat cancer exists in a patient and thyroid is affected at a later stage. Cancer capturing the thyroid gland may be less than one percent for which the reason is not known although some cases had been reported in the areas where radioactive activity took place (explosion to atomic bombs). Chernobyl region of Russia was one of them.

Regarding the classification of thyroid neoplasm (tumor), it may be noted that condition of thyroid can be *either benign or malignant*. A benign one is either papillary adenoma or follicular adenoma. The later is more common. In malignant cases, there are two stages, the primary and the secondary. In the primary category, it may be differentiated and undifferentiated carcinoma and further, if it is differentiated, it can be either papillary or follicular. Primary also has malignant lymphoma and medullary carinoma. In the secondary malignant stage, either it is metastatic (blood born or it is a local infiltration). Secondary growths of malignant tumors are rare. It is very difficult, rather impossible, to differentiate with absolute certainty between follicular adenoma and a follicular carcinoma because there is no evidence of capsular penetration. It is only after excision of an adenoma, that the follow up becomes clear for further line of treatment.

PATHOLOGY

The thyroid is found atrophied in most of the cases of hypothyroidism and as a result, it would weigh less than half the average. If the gland is not smaller in size, the histological examination reveals that the gland is composed, to a great extent, of fibrous tissue besides that the secretion of epithelium is diminished. This condition can also be called physiological atrophy where in the metabolism is also diminished and there are some qualitative changes including a considerable increase in the tolerance of dextrose.

SYMPTOMS

- The onset of the disease is slow and insidious.
- Weakness, lethargy, loss of memory and mental dullness of hebetudes. In *nervous system*, there is slowness of movement, delayed and impaired reflex activities. Electroencephalogram reflects decreased 'a' rhythm.
- Very sensitive to cold climate; needs more of bed covering and does not sweat or sweats little. The preference is for the warm room or weather.
- There is great dryness and roughness of *skin*. It has yellow waxy cast and it becomes thick, edematous due to deposition of myxematoes under the skin of whole body (myxematoes are semisolid materials, formed of sulphuric acid, proteins chondroitin and mucopolysaccharides). This causes disappearance of wrinkles. There may be flakes or fish-scale appearance of the skin. The nails also get brittle and dry while the hair get rough and dry. In some cases, the skin may get thickened but does not pit to pressure. It is harsh to touch. The sebaceous glands of the skin become inactive and the hair become dry, coarse and sparse. Falling of hair from the head is a common problem. Hair from outer canthus of the eyebrows fall out. The hands become clumsy and spade-like.
- *Muscle and joint* pains with special reference to shoulders and legs. Lumbago and rheumatism may be the chief complaints but rheumatism or neuritis in the joints may not have the characteristics features of rheumatism. The possibility in such

a case is hypothyroidism. The gait is uncertain and clumsy with muscular weakness.

- *Metabolism* is slow and the body temperature is on the lower side. BMR (*Basal metabolic rate*) is reduced to 30-45% below normal. Cold is poorly tolerated. Metabolism of fat, protein and carbohydrates are all below normal. The blood sugar tends to be on lower side of the normal range having increased tolerance of sugar. Cholesterol synthesis is increased along with fatty acid and phosphate mobilization whose values in the blood increases. On *minerals* side, there is a tendency to retain salts whereas on the vitamins side, conversion of beta-carotene to *vitamin* A is impaired. There is a rise in betacarotene level in the blood with carotinemia.
- *Constipation* exists due to reduced gastrointestinal motility and there is abdominal pain in rare cases. The appetite is poor.
- *Menstruation* is irregular and menometrorrhagia is there. There is increased menstrual flow, copious and prolonged with occasional amenorrhoea, sterility, habitual abortion, premature labor and foetal death.
- In *lactating women*, milk secretion fails.
- Vertigo, tinnitus, impaired hearing, chronic hoarseness of voice with a tendency to prolonged sinusitis.
- Puffiness of the eyes and extremities is common and it is uncomfortable too.
- Polyuria with nocturia and incomplete emptying of the bladder.
- Obesity inspite of diminished appetite and less of food intake.
- There is slowness of thinking power and speech with loss of concentration. Drowsiness and hallucinations.
- Under the neurological manifestations, the symptoms are deafness, headache with sleepy appearance, waxy and red colour of the cheeks (apple blossom cheeks). Tongue and lips are felt thick.

- Teeth may decay rapidly and could fall out as well.
- Heart sounds low, distant, muffled with a rate of 40 to 50 per minute. Tendency to arteriosclerosis. Heart is enlarged and flabby. With slow rate, the cardiac output is reduced to about 2.5 liter/minute. Electrocardiogram indicates low voltage ventricular complexes. There is not much changes in the blood pressure.
- In skeleton, not much change is observed.
- Anaemia is very common and the *blood* iodine level is low. Cholesterol level, fatty acids and phosphate levels are high in blood.
- Speech is slurring type, low tone and husky, and goes to the extent that sometimes it can be diagnosed over telephone.

The appearance of the patient suffering from hypothyroidism changes gradually. Although there is anorexia or loss of appetite yet in some cases, the weight puts on. Bloating feeling becomes usual and the rings on the fingers become tight showing thickening and puffiness of the body. One feels tired all the time and sheer exhaustion becomes a routine of the day. Depression and absentmindedness and mental sluggishness go on developing as the physical slowness progresses. The patient forgets the common past events and even the names of his/her friends. Everything one attempts to do appears to take an age. The most common feature of the disease is depression. *Sometimes, the patient is taken to a psychiatrist or a counsellor for treatment thinking it a mental disease which is not so, although many of the symptoms referred in depression or emotional disorder share common characteristics.*

CONNECTION WITH OSTEOPOROSIS

The disease of osteroporosis (bone-brittleness) has a positive connection with hyperthyroidism and hypothyroidism. It has a striking rate of about one in four women over the age of 60 and it is caused by *lack of calcium* in the bones. Some experts opine that it is due *to lack of collagen* in the connective tissues and the bones. *Collagen is a protein, which plumps up the cells in the bone and the skin.* In this condition of disease, the bones crush and fracture after great debility and pain is the first symptom and this leads to *Dowager's hump*, a disease showing symptoms of a bent back caused by small crush fractures in the spine. Bones break easily even on a small fall. It is well known that an overactive thyroid disturbs the calcium balance and the ability of the body to build strong bones. Now it is also known that patients with underactive thyroids or even normal thyroid profiles but having goiter are at the risk of developing osteoporosis especially when they are treated with T4. It has also been found by some research workers that there is about ten percent reduction of calcium in the forearm of sufferers who had been treated with T4 for over ten years and a four percent reduciton of calcium was found in those who were treated for more than five years of treatment. Some research workers also reported a significant decrease of bone mineral density in those women who were in their pre-menopausal or post-menopausal stage. They had a thinner bone structure in thighs, spine and forearms. It is also revealed by the research scholars that a chemical called Gla-protein was responsible for this. This is a sign of bone turnover in the blood of the women and discovered that much higher levels of Gla-protein was present in those women who were being treated with T4 than those who were normal. Such a study of bone mineral density also revealed an interesting fact that the patients had normal levels of thyroid hormones and thyroid function.

A careful monitoring of T4 is, therefore, essential on the part of the doctor so that a lowest dose is given to keep the thyroid functioning in normal state. Those suffering from bone disorder should get their blood checked regularly and maintain minimum suggested dose of T4 (a view).

The female-patient should also take care and stop smoking, if she smokes. She should conduct regular exercises. Brisk walk is one of them. Walking and dancing make the bones slightly mobile and help the bones to grow strong. Regular bone scan is needed at intervals to check the progress of bone density.

CLINICAL FEATURES

Although we have discussed about the symptoms of the disease yet it will be to benefit the readers to know the clinical features of hypothyroidism. If you find some repetition, please bear with me because the motive of writing clinical features is to make the subject clearer.

METABOLISM

BMR (Basal metabolic rate) is decreased to 30-45 percent below normal. The body temperature is on the lower tilt of the normal range and the patient cannot tolerate cold.

Metabolism of carbohydrates, proteins and fats are all below normal. The blood sugar is also on the lower side of the normal range with increased tolerance of sugar. Cholesterol is also increased along with fatty acid and phosphatids mobilization whose values increase in the blood. In the case of minerals, there is a tendency of the body to retain salts. Conversion of betacarotene level to vitamin A is impaired. There is a rise in betacarotene level in the blood with carotinemia.

APPEARANCE

The face is swollen, puffy patient, has no interest in seeing the surroundings and appears dull with a weary look. Hair from outer canthus of eyebrows fall out and hair of head are coarse and sparse.

SKIN

The skin of the patient is thick, dry and edematous due to depostion of myxematoes under the skin of whole of the body. Such a condition cause disappearance of wrinkles. The colour of skin is yellowish due to carotenemia.

ALIMENTARY TRACT

The prominent feature is anorexia and reduced gastrointestinal motility (moving power), which in turn leads to constipation.

SKELETON

There is no substantial change in the skeleton.

MUSCLES

Muscle tone is reduced. Jerks are also reduced in amplitude and delayed. The time of reaction is lengthened.

CARDIOVASCULAR MANIFESTATLIONS

There is not much of change in the blood pressure.

The heart is enlarged and blabby (without motive). The rate of heart beat is slow and the cardiac output is reduced (2.5 liter per minute). The ECG indicates low voltage ventricular complexes.

Cutaneous circulation. The skin is pale and cool as on vasodilation occurs.

GONADS

Not many histological changes are observed but failure of reproductive functions exists, which is induced by amenorrhea in woman, loss of libido and failure of fertility.

SECRETION OF MILK

In lactating women, the milk secretion stops.

NERVOUS SYSTEM

Delayed and impaired reflex activities with slowness of movements. Decreased 'a' rhythm, when checked on electroencephalogram.

BLOOD

Anaemic condition is common in hypothyroidism. The level of blood iodine is also low due to reduced iodine uptake by the thyroid. Cholesterol level of 400 to 700 mg per 100 ml is not unusual. Fatty acids and phosphatic levels are high in the blood.

SPEECH

The patient has a slow and husky voice. Some doctors are of the view that husky and slow voice is so much different that a good doctor can diagnose this clinical feature of the disease when talking over the phone with the patient.

PSYCHIC CHANGES

The patient will have lack of interest in the work, lack of concentration, initiative and mental activity, loss of memory and slow thinking. If prolonged under such conditions for a long time without any treatment, myxedema madness can develop in some subjects.

Difference Between Depression and Hypothyroidism

There is confusion on the part of the patient to differentiate between depression and hypothyroidism. It is difficult but can be judged with some keen interest taken by the patient. There are similarities of the symptoms too.

In the cases of *depression*, the following symptoms can be observed:

- The appetite increases.
- There is gradual weightloss.

HYPOTHYROIDISM MYXEDEMA

- Insomnia exists and the patient gets up early in the morning.
- Sleep is very less but the patient is not much worried about the quantum of sleep.
- A sense of inferiority complex or guilt.

In *hypothyroidism cases*, the following symptoms can be observed:

- There is adequate evidence of weight gain.
- The appetite is lost.
- Desires more of sleep, as the patient feels tired all the time.
- Impaired memory and slow thinking.

The common symptoms of depression and hypothyroidism are loss of interest in the work, in enjoying the pleasures of life and a sense of miserable feeling. It is the patient or his relative who should take interest to find out the difference between the two ailments. If by chance, doctor attending the patient also goes wrong and treats the hyperthyrodism taking the disease as a case of depression, the condition of the patient will go worse. The antidepressant drugs can dwindle the level of thyroid hormones and the side effects of antidepressant drugs may appear. These side effects are so common that it is difficult to judge them as side effects. These vary from dryness of mouth, sleepiness, blurred vision, constipation, nausea, sweating and trembling to rashes. Rashes on skin could be taken as positive sign for side effects of the drugs.

SUBJECTIVE SYMPTOMS

- Feels chilly with muscular weakness and aches.
- Gain of weight is noted.
- Slow in thinking and loss of concentration.
- A sense of depression overwhelms the patient.

- Nails are brittle and hair entangled easily, difficult to manage.
- Constipation becomes the prime symptom in some cases.
- Periods become irregular in appearance, delayed, earlier or prolonged.
- Headaches are common and eyelids are found sticky in the morning.
- Dyspnea is another feature. The patient is breathless.
- Frequent bouts of illness and infections with comparative slow recovery and healing.
- Tingling and numbness in the feet and hands are noted.
- Changes in the skin; thickness and pigmentation makes the patient worried.

WHAT THE PATIENT'S RELATIVE AND FRIENDS NOTE?

- Patient is observed pale with dry and puffy face.
- Coarse and dry hair is noted and hair loss is observed.
- Edema around the eyes is seen.
- Voice of the patient becomes husky and hoarse.
- More of snoring, if patient already snores. Starts snoring, if the patient did not have the habit of snoring earlier to the disease.
- Loss of interest in work by the patient. He or she does not enjoy the job, which he or she used to relish.
- A slight degree of deafness is also observed.

WHAT DOES THE DOCTOR NOTES?

- When the patient goes to the doctor, the disease is then diagnosed by some features like goiter, distention of the abdomen, delayed reply of questions, appearance as if the patient is lost somewhere, delayed reflexes, slow pulse rate, loss of muscle power and galactorrhoea (milk production even when not breast feeding in the case of women patients).

- If the patient is directed to outstretch his arm and hold out one finger in front of his face. The finger will show tremors. He will be nervous and reporting sleepless nights and a big appetite. Inspite of this, he will be losing weight. Such a condition is *hyperthyroidism.*
- On the other hand, if the patient is puffy faced and sluggish, it is *hypothyroidism.*
- *A good doctor will always go in for clinical tests to determine the disease. The blood sample will measure the amount of hormone hitchhiking on blood proteins. There have been a dozen tests developed and only a doctor can decide which are the best for the patient for prescribing.*

DIAGNOSIS

The disease comes insidiously and it is difficult to determine the accurate onset of the disease. There is a gradual diminution in the activity of the thyroid gland as the age advances. Impairment of memory and energy, loss of hair, and gain of body weight (provided the weight gain is not on account of an accumulation of fluid). All these symptoms lead to the pointer that hypothyroidism has caught hold of the body. An early sign is pain near the joints and in the joints. The limbs become thick but the skin does not pit on pressure. Following tests confirm:

- The basal metabolism may be estimated. Basal metabolic rate is lowered i.e. minus 14 to 15 percent.
- Butanol extractable iodine is lowered.
- Serum protein bound iodine lowered.
- Radio-active iodine uptake is low.
- Serum cholesterol level is high. It is usually more than 250 mg and sometimes touching as high as 800mg.
- In glucose tolerance test, the curve tends to be low and flat.

- Chest X-rays shows a large, flabby, atonic heart which means pericardial or pleural fluid.
- In Electrocardiography, there is bradycardia, prolonged TR intervals, changes in ST segments, T-waves of poor amplitude and frequently inverted.
- Urinary 17 - ketosteroids test is usually low, under 10 mg per 24 hours in men and under 5 mg per 24 hours in women.

DIFFERENTIAL DIAGNOSIS

- Pituitary myxedema.
- Chronic nephritis, which can be diagnosed by kidney function tests found to be altered in myxedema.
- Obesity.
- Coronay infarction and insufficiency.

When we talk of myxedema, there is need to understand the difference between *thyroid myxedema and pituitary myxedema.*

In thyroid myxedema, the serum cholestrol is raised, the sexual functioning is normal, there is no tumor or the like and radioactive iodine uptake is increased by about 7-8 percent, after TSH stimulation.

In pituitary myxedema, the serum cholesterol is normal in most of the cases, there is disturbance of inefficiency in the sexual funcitoning, the evidence of pituitary tumor exists and radioactive iodine uptake increases by 32.2 percent (average), while the normal value is 20.8 percent.

If the symptoms as stated above and the feelings are some indications, it is time to get the disease clinically confirmed by blood tests. This topic is left here because the procedure for diagnosis of hyperthyroidism is same and we shall know it when we go to *Hyperthyroidism* chapter of the book.

SECONDARY HYPOTHYROIDISM

What we have discussed above under the heading hypothyroidism is primary hypothyrodisim. In medical terms there exist another type of hypothyroidism in which the thyroid is not involved but the involvement is in the controlling gland pituitary or the hypothalamus in the brain. There may be abnormality in the production of thyrotropin releasing hormone (TRP) and this happens when there is some sort of hurdle in the conveying of messages between hormones and nerve cells. Here again there may be congenital defect in pituitary or hypothalamus or even development of some sort of cyst or tumor to make a hurdle.

So, there are basically two reasons for secondary hypothyroidism, the pituitary problems and hypothalamus problems.

GENERAL TREATMENT IN ALLOPATHY

Treatment of hypothyroidism in the allopathic system of medicine varies but mainly either of the following preparation is suggested to be given orally.

1. A reliable preparation of dried thyroid gland (desiccated thyroid).
2. L-Thyroxine (T4) is the official name and name of trade drug is Eltroxin tablet.
3. Laevo-thyroxine (T3) is the official name and name of trade drug are Cynomel and Tertroxin tablets.
4. Radioactive iodine.

There is a fixed dosage per day and as the time passes and conditions improve, minimum maintenance dose is prescribed. The medicine is supposed to be continued throughout the life but when the conditions improve after years of use, the medicine can be stopped as well.

When thyroid extract is badly borne or there is some other reasonable and adequate reason for another method of treatment, the doctors consider operation for thyroid; grafts are not available easily (Human thyroid having active secretions, fresh and undamaged).

Regarding the radioactive iodine, a cocktail of it is taken. Like ordinary iodine, it will find its way straight to thyroid and its radiation will start hammering the overproductive cells into submission. Radioactive iodine decays rapidly and hence virtually all radiation ceases within few weeks.

It is usually advised by the doctors in the allopathic system of medicines that the usual single dose of medicine prescribed for hyperthyroidism or hypothyroidism should be taken every day before breakfast. Once the dose is decided and one has started taking the medicine, he or she may feel some problems so long as one continues taking the medicine. Then there is a check up after, say, six weeks in which the blood is examined to see the levels of thyroid hormones. Thereafter, monthly checks are made till the symptoms of the disease are observed for a month or two. With the advance of medical science, the procedure as above has been simplified and monthly check are averted, if the symptoms of the disease do not correspond to earlier aggravated conditions. Usually the INMAS, (Institute of Nuclear Medicines) Timar pur, Delhi calls the patient after six months for check up. It is sort of trial of treatment.

If the condition does not improve *in the case of hypothyroidism*, the medicine will not be stopped. If the underactivity of thyroid is because of pituitary problems, the treatment will be made to correct the pituitary and then prescription will be made for T4. In occasional cases, when the under activity has affected the working of adrenal glands, the prescription of the doctor may detail steroids (hormones produced by the adrenals) until they are recovered.

If the thyroid gland has failed, one has to carry on taking T4 for the rest of life. It cannot be stopped for the rest of life till doctor advises. In case the medicine is discontinued, all the old symptoms of the disease will come back. As a matter of fact, half yearly check ups are essential to ensure the maintenance dose.

HOMOEOPATHIC TREATMENT FOR HYPOTHYROIDISM

In the case of goiter, there is apparent swelling seen on the neck but this may not be there in hypothyroidism. This is the reason there are many remedies for treatment of goiter but very few for hypothyroidism and hyperthyroidism. Symptoms which a body is presenting make a selection rather than the name of the disease.

It is difficult to pin point some specific remedy for this disease but few can be quoted for needful and serious study so that a rapid selection is made.

The great trio of Arg-n., Ars., and Nat-m.

This is the trio to be tried in case of this disease but it should be strictly followed in terms of symptoms - similarity and not as specific trio. In many cases, this trio has been tried and it has given success where the symptoms agreed. The trio is that of *Arg-n.*, *Ars.*, and *Nat-m*. Whenever you receive patients of hypothyrodism, check them, inspect them and surround them to see if they befit these three remedies before finally switching over to other related remedies in accordance with the symptoms. To help these trio is Tuberculinum bovinum, provided the patient has history of TB himself or herself or on the parent's side. There is no need that Tuberculinum should be given as an intermediate remedy with plenty of S.L. in between.

Think of these following remedies of the trio without significance to the name of the disease, hypothyroidism. The following symptoms of the remedies are based upon constitutional aspects with modalities to make them befit with the person.

Argentum nitricum

- If you make a scrutiny of the personality of the patient you are seeing, he or she looks older than the age written on your prescription card.
- If the patient is a woman, she has feeble features and looks dried up in disease.
- If it is a child, he or she will have looks of a withered old man.
- If the patient has been suffering from acute or chronic diseases from unusual or long continued mental exertion.
- If your patient complaints that as and when he or she starts for going outside the house for attending a party, picnic, conference, and important meeting, cinema, church, or a temple and even when starting a journey by car/train etc., there is an urge for stool. In some cases, two or three bouts of diarrhea are experienced.
- If the patient complains that his or her time passes very slowly.
- If the patient complains that he or she has a feeling as if the body or some part of the body is expanding.
- If the patient has noisy violent belching and complains of debility in the legs.
- If the patient craves for sugar and sweet food items.
- If the patient is chilly if uncovered, yet smothers (suffocates) when wrapped up.
- If the symptoms of the patient are worse at night and are ameliorated from cool air, cold drinks, and cold baths.
- If the symptoms of the patient appear on the left side of the body and patient craves fresh air.

Arsenicum album

- If the patient is chilly but he or she cannot define it because it is frequently intermingled with heat.
- If the patient gets better from heat.
- If there is a feeling of total insecurity and dependency on others.
- If there is burning with great restlessness and insatiable thirst. The patient drinks often but little at a time.
- If the aggravation of symptoms is after midnight, say 1 to 2 a.m. or even 1 to 2 p.m. in the afternoon.
- If the patient is very possessive, does not share relationship, does not believe in give and take, a selfish sort of person who believes in taking only.
- If the patient has fastidiousness. He or she is compulsively fastidious, wants to be neat and clean, desires every thing around him or her neat and clean in orderly manner. The cleanliness is to the point of expending inordinate energy, constantly cleaning and straightening.
- If the patient is very particular for his or her health only and has anxiety about his or her health. It is deep down inside, a fear of dying. In such a state he or she will try to exaggerate many symptoms even to the extent of blowing out the same.
- If the patient desires company. This desire is that he or she needs someone to be present near him or her. The patient surrounds himself or herself with people because of insecure sense concerning health.

Natrium muriaticum

- If the patient is emotionally sensitive and vulnerable but quite clear and strong on mental and physical levels. The patient has a high degree of objectivity and awareness with great responsibility to achieve or undertake objectives. Because of this, the patient lends a sympathetic ear to those of friends or relatives whom others avoid when in distress.

- If the patient is self-contained and solves his or her problem by himself. The patient does not want to hurt others nor does he likes to be hurt by others.
- If the patient has queer affections like falling in love with a married man, a driver or a neighbour knowing well that it is foolish and unwise to do so but cannot help it.
- If the patient is cachectic, anaemic, old, with catarrhal troubles and in case the patient is young, he has a tendency to grow fat.
- If the patient has a marked tendency to weep and all attempts to console him or her aggravate the state of mind, that is to say, aggravate the sadness and tearfulness and sometimes makes him angry too.
- If the patient wants to cry and be alone.
- If the patient has emaciation, more of body than of face. The collar-bones become prominent and the neck looks scrawny but the hips and lower limbs remain plump and round (Kent).
- If the patient loses flesh while living well. Face is pale, shining, greasy-looking, mapped tongue, violent thirst and sweats on face while eating. Corners of mouth are sore, cracked and crusty. Dryness of all the mucous membranes with coldness of many parts is associated.
- If the patient's mammary glands are wasted and lower extremities are dropsical with longing for salt.
- If the patient is a schoolgirl with bouts of anaemic headaches. Headaches, which appear periodically with great severity; head feels as if bursting. This may be chronic, periodical, semi-lateral and from sunrise to sunset. Headaches begin with partial blindness.
- If the patient has a pale face, nausea, vomiting. Most of the diseases occur between 10 a.m. and 3 p.m. and 5 p.m. to 7p.m.
- If the patient has an intolerance to heat, sensitive to light and is unable to pass urine or stool in the presence of others.

- If the patient has physical problems like gastritis, arthritis, migraine headaches, canker sores or herpes on the lower lips.
- If the patient is always washing or cleaning his or her hands. This fastidiousness is a fear of microbial contamination.
- If the patient has troublesome menstruation and her menses are too scanty or too late, too profuse or too soon.
- If the patient has aversion to bread, fat and rich things.
- If the patient has a long chain of mental symptoms; hysterical condition of the mind and body, weeping alternating with laughing; irresistible laughing at unsuitable times, prolonged, spasmodic laughter followed by tearfulness, great sadness, joylessness. (Kent)
- If the patient has a marked fluttering of the heart with intermittent and irregular pulse.

Calcarea carbonica

The remedy has been already discussed in the treatment of goiter and the readers may please refer to goiter chapter. However, when this remedy is indicated, the patient has cold damp feet, cold legs and night sweats. There is profuse sweat on the head during night and milk always disagrees. If it is a child, he or she has emaciated limbs and neck with malnutrition of glands, bones and skin. There is enlarged glands, emaciation of the neck and limbs while fat and the glands of the belly increase.

- Calc. patients gain weight easily and have difficulty in losing the weight even after low intake of calories.
- Another aspect of Calc. patient is that he or she is very lean and thin person with a cylindrical lean face with wrinkles over it. *This type of appearance is rare in Calc. patients but it cannot be ruled out that they are not so because they are not fat, soft, flabby or plump. The basic relation is resemblance of other Calc. symptoms.*

- They lack stamina and generally avoid physical activities. Over-exertion of the body is not tolerant to *Calc*. They are self reliant and withdrawn.
- They are usually constipated and feel better when their bowels get clear.
- They fear that they may have some infectious disease and always worry about their health. They fear about having serious diseases like cancer or heart failure. They even fear that they will die. They also have fear of thunderstorms and living in dark rooms.
- In a group of friends, *Calc.* person will cut silly jokes or keep on talking insignificant topics, which others may not like because those will not be of much importance to others.
- At times, they appear to lose their power of concentration and comprehension because they do not know what they desire.
- They are capable of hard work but spend hours to complete the jobs on hand because over-work tires them.
- They are surely intelligent but it is another aspect that their comprehension is a bit slow. It takes them time to understand the situation fully.

Tuberculinum

The remedy is deep acting, long acting, affects the constitution more deeply than other remedies. The patient has a longing for travel and always wants to go out of home. He or she is sensitive but dissatisfied. He has fear of dogs and avoids taking meat. He would rather like or crave for cold milk. He may have shining hair and very blue sclerotic lips. Patients of *Tuberculinum* patient have excessive sweat and chronic diarrhea and are driven out of bed with diarrhea. They feel better when they ride an open vehicle scooter, bike etc. where cold wind must strike them. If the climate is damp cold, they do not like so.

- Tuberculinum patient is unpredictable in his or her mood and behaviour. They will be very soft spoken one minute and speak harsh the other moment. They are never satisfied with themselves and feel that their life is short.
- They are difficult people to live with because of their contradictory behaviour, aggressiveness and selfish nature. They always desire self-gratification but do not attain it.
- They always seek a change not for places or traveling but in their jobs also. They will leave one job and get another. Once they find a problem in one situation, they will seek another place to find a solution. According to one scholar, their traveling is not a desire but a compulsion. They are driven to it.
- In sex, they appear to be hyperactive. They have strong sexual desires to the extent that they would not hesitate to change one partner to another. Their love affairs have a sort of commotion and conflict.
- They have a desire for fat and ice cream, perspire heavily and particularly at night in bed. Their whole body is drenched in sweat, which is also offensive and they have to change their socks frequently.
- They have a fear of dogs and cats. Fear for cats is so immense that a doctor can give this remedy blindly if he finds the patient having fear of cats. The patient not only fears the cat but also does not want to touch it and has disgust for it. Probably they get allergy with the fur of cats and dogs.
- *Tuberculinum* should not be given as a routine. The patient must have a family history of tuberculosis. After confirming this, other symptoms as detailed above must be verified before induction of this remedy.

VIEWS OF GEORGE ROYAL

George Royal in his book, 'Homoeopathic Theory and Practice of Medicine' has given a comprehensive data about hypothyroidism. This sums up all the data given earlier in different modes above while discussing about this disease. The readers would like to study the following:

"The skin of the face shows the first manifestations, viz., swollen, firm, inelastic, dry and rough. This gives the face a peculiar expression i.e., broad, bulky, coarse, stupid, almost imbecile; this is especially true of the congenital form, i.e., cretins. The skin becomes dry, the nails brittle and the hair fall out. The bulk of the body enlarges, especially in the region of neck, though the thyroid gland may be smaller or absent. Edema may be present but does not pit as in the edema due to renal insufficiency; the tissue of the lips, nose and tongue is thickened. The voice becomes slow, monotonous, co-ordination becomes impaired, slowing the movement of the body. All the mental perceptions are dulled, and the senses changed, taste, smell etc. At first, the patient may be irritable then come delusions, hallucinations, etc., ending in dementia; temperature and metabolism are lowered. Ascites is present in some cases, also hemorrhage from any tissue or organ. The thyroid gland is not palpable due to the changes in the muscles of the neck.

Diagnosis is scarcely ever mistaken for any other disease.

Prognosis: The prognosis is very favorable in all cases except those in which the functions of the glands have been suddenly destroyed by any disease or surgery.

CRETINISM — FETAL OR INFANTILE HYPOTHYROIDISM

Cretinism is a synonym of hypothyroidism *but it has a different starting time.* It is a condition of hypothyroidism starting in fetal or early childhood/infancy. While making a study on disorders of hypothyroidism in the beginning of the topic under hypothyroidism, we have discussed about cretinism. Let us make a brief recollection of the same. Sporadic (singly or scattered instances) cretinism is a complete or near complete failure of thyroid gland development. In such a case, the parents of the child will be normal in thyroid functioning. In the areas where cretinism is more or we can say in endemic areas, cretinism with goiter is a common feature and it is due to maternal reasons and total iodine deficiency. The child with goitrous cretinism will be pot-bellied, having umbilical hernia, protruding tongue and pale puffy face. In adolescence and adult age, the patient is physically and mentally retarded. He or she will have dry, wrinkled skin and supraclavicular pads of fat.

In most of the cases, symptoms of cretinism are manifested after six months of age because the child gets sufficient amount of hormones through mother's milk when he or she is on breast feed. The most common cause is iodine deficiency and if the disease is diagnosed early, the treatment is possible, otherwise once the features and the outcome of the disease are established nothing can be done.

SYMPTOMS AND SIGNS IN EARLY CHILDHOOD

The child suffering from this disease shows no interest in playing, has lack of vitality, is restless and suffers from constipation, his or her normal body activities are limited because he or she has no interest or initiative to do any thing. He or she has low resistance and hence prone to various infections which overpowers him or her from time to time.

DELAYED DEVELOPMENT AND OTHER ACTIVITIES

- The child does not gain weight or height as he or she should with progressive months.

- The dentition, which should take place by fifth or sixth month, is delayed considerably.
- In the third month, child should hold up the head and sit but it is also delayed.
- The child should have closed fontanelle (bones of vertex) by sixth months or so. He or she should be able to stand, make speech but in cretinism, all these action are delayed.
- The child should walk by one or one and half years of age but this is also delayed.
- Even after the child learns to stand, his or her erect posture is not perfect and one can see that the child is dwarfish. His or her fingers are short and club shaped and bones/teeth are deformed.
- The growth of the muscles and skeleton is less. The child has a large tongue in small mouth. The face has a look of an idiot. The lips are thick and saliva dribbles from it. The nose has a broad shape with bridge depressed.
- The child has thick, coarse and dry skin on which wrinkles appear. There is irregular deposit of fat in the body and excessive deposition is seen above the clavicle.
- The child has subnormal intelligence and looks dull.
- In some cases, the child is deaf and mute.
- The appetite of the child is less and gastrointestinal mobility is low which in turn leads to constipation. The abdomen is distended with gases and the child is pot-bellied.
- On blood side, his PBI content is low, cholesterol is high and sugar tolerance is increased with low blood glucose level.
- On nervous signs, the child has defect in speech and difficult orientation of place or time. The coordination is defective, sensation is dull and motor function is below par. Reflexes are sluggish and delayed.

- On metabolic side, his or her BMR is low by twenty to forty percent of the normal child of his or her age.

TREATMENT

As it has been detailed, cretinism cannot be controlled once the signs appear and it is futile to do anything. When early signs are observed in a child, it is better to keep the child warm by daily massaging of the body. It is sometimes useful. Lack of development of thyroid gland or partial development of thyroid cannot be helped by medicines. The treatment is not likely to do much when without thyroid but can supplement its action efficiently at least in homoeopathy. Cretinism has been successfully treated in many cases where the thyroid is functioning partially and the child is in the infancy stage. Considering the symptoms, one can start the treatment. *Bar-c.* has been found most useful in the beginning as most of the symptoms of this remedy coincide with the children suffering from cretinism. Delayed speech, delayed dentition, delayed standing and sitting are all covered by this remedy and I have personally treated few patients, who had their simultaneous treatment from A.I.I.M.S., New Delhi. This allopathic treatment was not stopped and the only medicine given to them was *Bar-c.* [(Please see page 91 for more remedies on the subject)]. There was some improvement in their stature and intelligence. Complete cure of this disease is not possible.

Hyperthyroidism— Thyrotoxicosis

HYPERTHYROIDISM as the name suggests is the opposite of hypothyroidism. An exophthalmic goiter, Parry's disease, *Grave's disease* or Basedow's disease, all are the synonyms of hyperthyroidism. It is a condition of the thyroid in which the size of the gland increases and there is abnormal secretion of thyroid stimulating hormone. Loss of weight, tremors of hands, palpitation and speedy action of the heart, general debility and nervous irritability are the other manifestations of this disease. Abnormal or overproduction of thyroid hormones is reasoned by the overactive thyroid gland. It is easy to detect this overaction of the gland than the underactive thyroid. Here again, females suffer more than the males; it is usually in early adult life. The onset of the disease is most commonly in between the age of 15 to 30 years. Hereditary factor cannot be ruled out here also. Hypothyroidism slows down the action of body's metabolism but hyperthyroidism is reverse of it. It increases the metabolism of the body.

If a *definition of hyperthyroidism or thyrotoxicosis* is to be made, it can be said that it is a condition on account of abnormal secretion of the thyroid gland in which the size of thyroid is increased. There will be loss of weight, slight tremor of the hands, protrusion of eyes, palpitation or rapid action of the heart and general debility or nervous irritability. A more clear definition can be as follows:

Hyperthyroidism is linked with hypersecretion of thyroid hormones along with numerous clinical manifestations defined by weight loss, increased BMR and sensitivity to tremors, increased vascularity of the gland and also goiter exophthalmos.

It is of two types, primary thyrotoxicosis and secondary thyrotoxicosis:

1. *Primary thyrotoxicosis* is a syndrome characterized by hyperactivity of the thyroid gland associated with excessive production of thyroxine. When hyperthyroidism is associated with goiter and ocular signs, it is said to be Grave's disease or Basedow's disease or Parry's disease.
2. *Secondary thyrotoxicosis* is the condition when hyperthyroidism is associated with *nodular* goiter.

ETIOLOGY

The disease of hyperthyroidism is common in hot countries than in cold countries and of course civilized races are more prone to this disease. Family predisposition cannot be ruled out but it is not evident that the disease is hereditary. There have been different observations about the males and females affected with this disease but according to some observers, the ratio of females and males is 6:1 and the common age of this disease is between 15 and 30 years. The disease is an autoimmune disorder. *(Adams and Purves* (Research Scholars) first isolated LATS (Long acting thyroid stimulator) from the serum of thyrotoxic patients and this is now accepted to be responsible for this disorder. It is immunoglobulin in nature and is liberated from the lymphocyte.

Here are few more causes:

- More than needed secretion of thyroid stimulating hormone.
- More than needed sensitivity of the thyroid follicles to

thyroid stimulating hormones as we find in staphylococcal infection.
- Psychological trauma like accidents, fright, emotional disturbance or shock, severe and prolonged illness.
- Genetic predisposition.

CAUSES OF OVER ACTIVITY OF THYROID

The causes for the hyperthyroidism are three major and five rare as follows:

Major causes
- Grave's disease (Autoimmune system reacting to own tissues as foreign).
- Plummer's disease (Toxic multinodular goiter).
- Toxic adenoma (Benign non cancerous lump).

Rare causes
- Excess production of iodine of Jod-Basedow disease.
- Post-partum thyroiditis (after the birth of a child).
- Thyrotoxicosis factitia (addiction of thyroid hormones).
- Some problems with the pituitary gland.
- Silent thyroiditis.

Major causes

1. Grave's disease

The most common or general cause of the disease is Grave's disease. It is almost seven or eight out of ten cases. It is an autoimmune condition like Hashimoto's disease in which immune system reacts as if its own tissue were foreign. Naturally, it has a family background and family immune system in which a group of genes are responsible. This disease is common in the ages between

20 and 40 years but can involve even babies as young as five or six years. Grave's disease is the name given by doctors of USA and UK whereas in Europe, this disease is also named as *Basedow's* disease after a German doctor's name.

Sir *Robert Graves* first coined the term *Grave's disease* in the early 19th century. It is one of the most common diseases of thyroid gland and a major cause for hyperthyroidism. It is a condition in which the thyroid gland produces excessive hormones. Once it is treated with medication, it may disappear for a few months and then again come back. If it is left untreated, it can lead to serious complication—even death. This disease does cause some discomfort but has no long-term adverse health consequences, if the patient gets proper treatment in time.

We know that the hormones produced by thyroid gland control the metabolism. Metabolism has a direct link to the amount of hormones that circulate in the blood stream. The metabolism will be overactive if the thyroid gland secretes more hormones due to some reason and this will cause pounding heart condition, sweating, trembling and weight loss. These are the symptoms of hyperthyroidism. Generally, the order for production and release of thyroid stimulating hormone (TSH) is made by pituitary gland in the brain. With overactive metabolism, there are false signals and overproduction of hormones take place. Why the immune system begins to produce these aberrant antibodies is unclear and we are going to discuss about this now.

A general view of the experts about *Grave's disease* is that there is *genetic fault* in the functioning of suppressor T cells, which inhibit activity of order cells undertaking immune response. If such a theory is accepted, the antibodies against the areas of the membrane of the thyroid cells are produced. These cells have TSH receptors, which makes the thyroid to grow and reproduce T3 and T4. There are other antibodies also like long acting thyroid stimulator (LATS) and LATS protector, which block TSH from binding to the membrane of thyroid gland.

How these antibodies arise or come from is another question? According to one theory, thyroid cells themselves have *faulty TSH receptors* and it is this faulty TSH, which triggers the production of thyroid stimulating antibodies resulting in overproduction of thyroid hormones. *Faulty immune mechanism* is another theory in which the body fails to recognize the antibodies as being harmful in their potential. Some experts present another theory that the cause of the overproduction of hormones is due to *food poisoning* but no concrete evidence is available on this aspect.

Stress also has been a main culprit not only in thyroid diseases but in many other diseases too. This reason cannot be ruled out. In a number of diseases, our immune system becomes weak by mental conditions like tension, overwork, anxiety, fear, exhaustion and fright. The possibility of attacking the thyroid by tension is almost accepted because the emotional turmoil is the fore-runners of thyroid disease. A lot of research has been done in the past over this issue and there are different views about tensions attacking the thyroid. A nineteenth century physician, Robert James Graves of Dublin, UK was the first who made a connection of overactive thyroid gland together with goiter with that of tensions. In a paper published by him in 1835, he reported this after experimenting with his patients. It is his name that indicates the name of disease, Grave's. Another physician, Caleb Hillier Parry later confirmed the view of Grave and was one of the first to agree on this. In 1991, Swedish doctors further put this aspect on research and they suggested that long-term anxiety, unhappiness and other negative feelings could be a possible factor for the disease. A surprising outcome of this research brought out another aspect for this disease. Prior to the thyroid disease, many people were found to have suffered from minor infections like colds and cystitis in the years previous to the attack of thyroidism. According to them, stress was one cause but the infections, rather frequent infections, lower the immune system and that is how the immune system gets weakened. Weak immune system along with tensions, causes the likelihood of the disease catching the roots of the body i.e. Grave's disease.

The amazing part of this research is that the theory of infections hampering the immune system can be vice versa. *If the Grave's disease has already occurred due to reasons other than infections, the immune system becomes weak and the patients are more susceptible to minor infections.*

However, all this discussion does not say that the stress is to be blamed for triggering Grave's disease but it does suggest that *stress is one of the important factors to either start the disease or maintain the disease.* One of the indecisions in concluding the causes in respect of which is first, the Grave's disease or the infections is that the disease comes so insidiously that the picture become unclear. It is never clear whether the stressful events came before or after the true onset of disease or whether the disease is more emotionally or physically linked?

2. Plummer's disease

Plummer's disease known as *toxic multinodular goiter* is a common disease in older women. In this disease, the overacting thyroid causes the existing goiter to become irregular and lumpy in shape or we can call it nodular. Nodular goiter is due to shortage or excess of iodine in the body, which could be due to diet or some drugs affecting the goiter formation. Erratic over stimulation on the part of the thyroid by TSH (the thyroid hormone) produced by the pituitary is sometimes the cause. Thyroid in such a case may be normal in its functioning but the nodules may become over active. This over activity is what we call multinodular goiter.

3. Toxic Adenoma

If the over activity is caused by a single nodule, such a condition is called as toxic adenoma or hot adenoma. It is a benign, non-cancerous lump, which is common in middle aged persons or persons in the later life. The belief is that the cause relates to increased iodine intake by the persons. A lump in the body puts the patient in extreme anxiety and worry and he or she jumps to the name of cancer. It may be taken as almost granted that such lumps are not cancerous or malignant. To confirm, whether it is cancerous, some tests confirm this by needle biopsy, if it is solid. If it is a cyst, filled with fluid, composition of the nodule can be determined.

Rare causes

1. Jod-Basedow disease or excess of iodine

Both shortage of iodine and excess production of iodine in the body can become a cause of thyroid disease. Excess of iodine is in particular those cases where the patient already suffers from a thyroid disease. The result is severe type of hyperthyroidism. Such a condition is also known as Jod-Basedow disease.

2. Post-partum thyroiditis

Less than five percent of all cases of thyroiditis in women are after childbirth which makes them prone to hyperthyroidism. It is during the period of pregnancy that immune system slows down to prevent the body reject the baby as a 'foreign' object. If the women are already suffering from hyperthyroidism, the autoimmune system has a tendency to improve in the late stages of pregnancy but this reverts to its original path after the baby is born. Those women who are not suffering from any disease of the thyroid also can get some disturbance of thyroid activity. This condition is known as *post-partum thyroiditis*. This may be a nodular goiter or simply an inflammation of the thyroid. Such a condition generally comes after two or three months of the childbirth and most of the times it is overactivity of the thyroid. After four to seven months of the birth of baby, over activity may be followed by under activity of the thyroid. Further after some time such a condition also goes away and the woman is normal. There are instances when the woman exclusively experience over-active phase of the disease and not the under active phase at all. The condition can be reverse also when only under active phase is felt and not the over active phase. According to survey of endocrinologists, as many as four out of ten women, who get hypothyroidism after the birth of child, get permanent thyroid failure by the end of baby's first year. Another two out of ten women get hypothyroidism after three or four years of childbirth.

It is really difficult to diagnose the disease at the stage after the birth of child. There are common features like weakness, fatigue, lack of energy, dry skin and falling of hair and depression in case the child is a female, especially in India. Such features are always reported in the clinics. The husbands and mother in laws of the woman who has given a birth to a child, be it son or daughter, do not act seriously upon the reporting of the woman about above complaints. They always feed her more of fat/protein diet generally accepted in Indian families ignoring the other aspect of thyroidism. In educated families, the post natal depression connection with the women due to *birth of a female* is faded away once the baby starts its childlike activities in the home but in middle and poor class of families, the in-laws go on cursing the women thus increasing the depression and in turn, the thyroidism. Post partum thyroiditis (PPT) can develop due to above reason along with other reasons like strained relationship of husband and wife, domestic problems, housing problems due to small flats (after the birth of another member of the family), or even history of emotional turmoil. If such emotional upsets are solved, the PPT can be avoided to some extent.

The surprising part of the episode is that the physician also does not take the things so seriously and perhaps needs a second opinion of clinical tests for which the guardians of the woman are not ready psychologically. They would like to wait for a few months after the birth of child than to accept the doctor's advice. In most of the cases, the disease goes away of its own, if it is post-partum thyroidism (hereafter PPT) and not concerned with Grave's disease. Grave's disease on the other hand needs proper treatment. *Another aspect of this PPT, which goes away on its own, is that it can return after the birth of second, third or fourth child.* Those who can afford and are well conversant with PPT take proper care to keep a watch through doctor's paraphrenalia and take action before the birth of next child but it is really an uncommon feature practically. If there is a note recorded regarding PPT on the medical discharge tickets of the woman giving birth to her first child (child born in modern maternity homes), it can be pointed out by the husband of the woman when she goes in for her second childbirth so that the doctors can take proper measures.

Now we come to very important measures, which the women can adopt after the delivery cases. It is but natural that the women get upset after they see their figure uneven after the birth of child. The second is scars on the abdomen region but these depressions along with other reasons of depression can be easily overcome.

Women can help avoid PPT childbirth by following measure:

- In Indian set up of families, half of the depression is gone *when the child is a male.* The modern educated families now ignore this attitude of difference of gender and it is not a cause of depression anymore. One is helpless in this regard and should accept the precious gift of God in any form. In spite of the husband accepting the gift gladly (he is more attached to the girl gift than the mother), some mothers blame themselves, which is wrong. Mothers should accept the gender happily and gracefully and thereby avoid depression.

- The women who still cry or get angry over the above issue after the birth of child, let it be any reason, should be allowed to cry and weep in silence. Sometimes, such crying or weeping gives relief to the emotional upsets developed within.

- After the child is four to six months of age, husband and wife should visit their relatives and friends so that the long detention of wife, confined to bed or her house, get relief and outlet of emotional feelings.

- Husband should encourage his wife to go for walks in the morning, do some exercise, resort to aerobics or dancing classes, and join some health clubs so that she restores her original figure.

- If the woman is lonely living without the in-laws, it is better that she keeps some good music cassettes of her liking near her bed so that she can listen to songs of her liking when alone. TV viewing is another time passing factor provided it is used within a limit.

- Women who have a literary mind and like to read books should be encouraged to read the literature of their liking.

- Any hobby, which gives a satisfaction to the woman after the birth of child should be resorted to. It may be painting, sewing, swimming, or creative writing and this should be given some time.

- Women who cannot afford to leave their houses for a walk outside due to paucity of time and domestic bindings, it is better to resort to 'Yoga', which can be learnt from an expert and carried out at home. This gives a good relief to PPT.

- Those who believe in the prayers to God and like to visit temples, gurudwaras, mosques or churches, should be encouraged to do so. Faith itself is a great healer in PPT. As a matter of fact, I have seen many families visiting the holy place of their faith immediately after the birth of child. The child is specially taken to the temple and blessed by the priests.

- Perhaps taking PPT into account, many of our religious ceremonies like "chola", "Janau, the sacred thread", "naming the child", "Anna-prasann" and performing "Hawan" (lighting sacred fire and prayers) are continuing since times immemorial. Every faith has different name to these ceremonies and I have mentioned a few. In any case, such ceremonies should be performed and never missed. This is a very good out-burst for encaged emotional feelings during pregnancies and birth of children.

PATHOLOGY

Pathology of the disease, perhaps, is most complicated subject in the history of medicine. There is lot of research going on for this. Thyroid is a derivative of a comparatively simple body called trihydrotriiodo-oxybetaindolpropionic acid, named thyroxine by its isolator. Again, this is not the only important substance. If an injeciton of thyroxine is given in the blood stream, it does not cause tachycardia unless amino acids are in the blood. This means that there is a scope of possibility that thyroxine is a derivative of a more complex body, which is less stable. Even if we consider that thyroxine is the cause of symptoms of the disease, we have to keep in mind as to what is the reason that leads to excessive production. It is seen that repeated stimulation of the sympathetic nerves to the thyroid leads to symptoms of hyperthyroidism but stimulation of sympathetic nerves may be made by the suprarenal glands or by toxins of the alimentary tract. Now when we consider the former as reason for stimulation i.e. suprarenal, we must remember that the disease will be of emotional origin. In the later case i.e. alimentary, the disease could be considered as due to infection.

So, the whole matter is confusion so far. Some medical experts say that under such confusion, exophthalmic goiter should not be called hyperthyroidism because the disease is due to qualitative change in the secretion and not due to quantitative change.

SYMPTOMS

- Extreme *nervousness*, fear, restlessness, anxiety, irritability, excitability, emotional instability, speech defects and temper alternating with weeping in women.
- Loss of *weight* despite voracious appetite and excellent food intake.
- *Tremors* while holding a cup of tea or tremulous sensations inside. It is one of the cardinal manifestations. Hypotonia and myopathy (any disease of muscle) may also be noted.
- Palpitations and pounding heart action, *dyspnea* and angina on slight exertion, *edema of face*.
- An unpleasant feeling of *warmth*, the patient desires less clothing during day and does not want covering at night, the perspiration is more, the skin is mostly moist and there may be *pruritus* too in some cases.
- Specific *weakness* of some muscles especially legs even on least exertion, which may be due to potassium depletion.
- Polydipsia, polyphagia and occasional diarrhea. The diarrhea is unexplained and there is discomfort in abdomen with epigastic pain stimulating gastric ulcers in some cases.
- *Swelling* in the front of neck (Goiter). This may be uneven, lumpy or smooth and symmetrical. The skin may be red and puckered. In some cases, the fingers show clubbing.
- Continued progressive *bulging of eyeballs*, unusually bilateral, increased lachrymation and photophobia may occur prior to signs *(exophthalmos)*. In this condition called exophthalmos, there is widening of the palpebral fissure and the upper eyelid partly covers the upper margin of the cornea. When the patient stares ordinarily, the whole of cornea is not exposed but in the case of exophthalmos, the whole of cornea is exposed due to retraction of the upper eyelids. The protrusion of the eyeballs

is due to retro-orbital edema and deposition of fat in the orbital cavity.

[Eye problems in the form of inflamed and swollen eye muscles and tissues can cause the eyeballs to protrude from the sockets. This is a specific complication of Grave's disease. It is also a fact that only a small percentage of Grave's patients experience this condition of protrusion of eyeballs. Those who get this protrusion do not generally denote serious problems of eyes. The eyes may have feeling of dryness, aching and irritation and probably this is due to the fact that eye lids can no more protect the eyes effectively from sunlight and injuries due to protrusion of eye balls. In very severe cases of eye protrusion, although a rare phenomenon, swollen eye muscles can put heavy pressure on the optic nerve resulting in even partial blindness. Eyes muscles weakened by longer periods of inflammation can lose their ability to control movement, which in some cases leads to diplopia or double vision of objects.]

- *Diminished menstrual flow*, both in quantity and duration. In severe cases of thyrotoxicosis, oilgomenorrhea and amenorrhea both occur in more than fifty percent of cases. Menorrhagia is rare. In *males, impotence* is reported in about 30 percent of cases.

- Pulse rate and the heart rate are increased and also the same persists in sleep thus making it different from funcitonal tachycardia. Those patients who are in young age suffer from a persistent tachycardia accentuated by exercise and emotions. The persons who are older are prone to paroxysms of tachycardia either in regular rhythm or with auricular fibrillation. (about ten percent cases). This symptom can lead to heart failure but is rarely associated with thyrotoxicosis. There is increase in pulse pressure. The pulse is collapsing in character. There is instability of the vasomotor system with flushing of face and neck.

- Talking of *metabolism*, there is increased basal metabolic rate, which results in canine hunger but at the same time, there is weight loss. Bones do not get demineralized as can be seen in radiography.

DIAGNOSIS AND GENERAL OBSERVATIONS

- The patient looks ill, his or her speech is rapid, a sense of stupor, anxiousness; tense and tremulous with loss of weight. Skin is warm, flushed and moist and thyroid is enlarged. The heart rate is rapid, may be 100-130 per minute, heavy pulsation visible, heart beats with loud snapping first sound at the apex with occasional systolic thrill and murmur. Rhythm of heartbeat is usually regular.
- Fine tremors when arms are out stretched and fingers extended. General body tremors as if from inside and exaggerated deep reflexes are observed.
- Blood pressure is lightly elevated and there is tendency of low-grade fever, say from $99.6°$ to $100°$ F in the afternoon.
- Exophthalmos or prominence of eyes can be seen. This can be checked as follows:
  - If the patient is told to see the finger of the doctor by keeping his/her sight on the finger put in front of his eyes, the lid will go very slow or lag when the finger is moved downwards. This condition in exophthalmos is called *Graefe's sign*.
  - If the convergence is poor, it is *Mobius sign*.
- Sleeping pulse rate is above 90 per minute in the absence of other casues.

GENERAL VIEW ABOUT THE PATIENT

In some patients of hyperthyroidism, there is a change in his/her *thirst*. There may be lot of thirst with passing of urine in large quantity, just like experienced in diabetics. The over activity of the thyroid could disturb centers in the brain that control the thirst threshold. This sort of complaint or disturbance appears to be linked to the secretion of vasopressin hormone, which causes the kidneys to retain water and prevent excessive water being passed as urine. On the other hand, this thirst and urine has direct link with anxiety and tension factor responsible in thyroidism.

There is swinging of the *mood of the patients* from joy to anxiety to depression and so on. If you have noted in the description given in hypothyroidism, the symptoms therein are often attributed to depression and it is mistaken as a psychological problem. In hyperthyroidism, depression may be seen as a cause rather than the effect of the problem. As a matter of fact, before depression and anxiety is taken as granted for hypo or hyperthyroidism, it is better to confirm the disease by tallying with other symptoms of the disease.

The *appearance* of the patient suffering from hyperthyrodisim is changed. The skin turns hot, pink, thin and moist. They flush easily. Palms are sweaty and have reddish looks. Their hair get thin and tend to fall off and nails also become thin or flaky. All the skin symptoms tend to go to the thinner side.

Some patients develop *tremors* in their fingers most of the time, when the hand is stretched out. This can be attributed to the over sensitivity to the stress hormone, adrenalin.

There are *changes in the eyes*. Eyes are always a tell tale tool in diagnosing a disease. The patient will go on staring without responding. There may be swelling around the eyes and may cause bags under the eyes or show swollen eyelids. Problems of focussing the object or even double vision cannot be ruled out. *Bulging of eyes* is mostly associated with the disease but this is uncommon and according to an estimate only one in twenty patients have such problems along with other complications of the eyes. Those who experience severe eye problems and bulging of eyes are the worst sufferers of this disease.

Goiter is another associate of this disease and it has its association with hypothyroidism too. A short introduction is given here but we shall discuss goiter in the forthcoming chapters. Goiter can be observed as severe swelling or slight fullness in the neck. In the former case, it is difficult for the patients to even close the top buttons of the shirt or wear an old chain earlier fitting to the patient. There is a variation of goiter in some patients. This variation is that goiter is very smooth in texture and soft to touch with rich blood vessels. When the patient puts his finger on the smooth skin of the goiter, he or she can feel the blood rushing through it. When the doctors puts his stethoscope over it, he can hear the blood surging turbulantly through the vessels. It is a sound, which is called *'thyroid bruit'* (A bruit is a sound in the arteries or veins when circulation of blood is at an abnormal speed).

Hyperthyroidism or over activity of the thyroid can disturb the metabolism connected with *calcium level*. If the calcium level in the body is low, there is a risk of catching *osteoporosis,* and muscle and *bone weakness.*

The over activity of thyroid has another disorder to its credit and that is *palpitation*. Acceleration of the pulse rate, palpitation and an irregular heart-beat is common for those patients who catch this *disease in the middle or old age*. Such cases are sometimes wrongly diagnosed as heart disease. In the same manner, breathlessness is also one of the features of the disease in some cases and it is also misdiagnosed as asthma or bronchitis.

WHAT DOES THE PATIENT FEELS?
- A feeling of warmth and heat, and moist palms.
- Excessive sweating.
- Nervousness, anxiety and excitabilty.
- Loss of sleep, insomnia, crowding of thoughts.
- Palpitation and weight loss.
- Increased appetite.
- Dry skin, flushes easily and hair loss.

- Goiter.
- Increased hunger for sex.
- Loss of muscle strength, weak muscles.
- Eye complaints and staring eyes.

WHAT THE PATIENT'S RELATIVES AND FRIENDS NOTE?
- Change of mood in the patient while talking.
- Talkative and boastful.
- Agitate on slightest provocation.
- Weight loss.
- Change of appearance like swollen neck, staring eye.
- Trembling and shaking in the extremities.
- Change of skin texture.

WHAT DOES THE DOCTOR NOTE?
- Low blood pressure.
- Tremors of extremities.
- Pulse is fast.
- Heartbeat is irregular.
- Reflexes are brisk.

ALLOPATHIC LINE OF TREATMENT

First of all, the patients should not take iodine containing drugs or antithyroid drugs. In general measure, the patients should be advised to take a short period of rest, especially if he or she suffers from congestive cardiac failure. In other cases, the patient is tackled in the outdoor lobby of the hospital. The patients have to be assured that they would be all right and his/her relatives should look into their personal problems based upon psychological factors. Such a tackling gives a dramatic relief to the patient.

If the things are not favorable on the mental side, some doctors prescribe sedative too, which show good results at time.

Diet should be quite liberal and of high calorie value.

Blockers and antithyroid drugs are the specifics in most of the cases.

Partial thyroidectomy (subtotal) is also done removing about seven-eighth of the gland leaving free the upper and lower poles.

Radioactive iodine and X-ray irradiation are also resorted to.

The first step by the doctor is that he has to make sure it is Grave's disease and for this he conducts one or two tests although he has option to conduct more tests to confirm the disease after initial tests. An analysis of the blood taken from the patient will show levels of two hormones, *thyroxine and triiodothyromine*, which are regulated by the thyroid. If they are higher then normal and if the level of TSH in the blood is abnormally low, the patient has *hyperthyroidism* and Grave's disease is the culprit.

To check whether there are large quantities of iodine collecting in the thyroid, a radioactive iodine uptake test is needed. This indicates that the gland requires large quantity of iodine to produce thyroid hormones and so if it is absorbing unusually large amounts of iodine, it is producing too much hormones.

In case, there is swelling of eyeballs or protrusion of eyeballs and that is the only visible symptom, the doctor will go in for hyperthyroidism tests although it may not be there and the reason may be problems in the eye muscles exclusively. For this the doctor may go in for VAT, MRI and ultrasound tests.

The objective of the treatment is to restore thyroid hormone level and to relieve discomfort. The treatment of hyperthyroidism is a little more complicated than that of hypothyroidism. Patience is required since the treatment may linger on for months or may take a year or more for symptoms to subside. The conditions of

HYPERTHYROIDISM—THYROTOXICOSIS

the disease revert at times after antithyroid drugs are taken. Attacks of the disease occur and hence a long term treatment lies ahead. The first duty of the doctor under the allopathic system of medicine is to use antithyroid drugs. In many cases, the patients get their thyroid restored to normal functioning.

The problem is that the drugs do not bring about a permanent cure. One has to remember that one has to take the medicines regularly without fail and one should also be ready to make periodical visists to the doctor to know the condition of the thyroid. The exact or precise line of treatment varies from doctor to doctor. Patient should know the stages of treatment for his own knowledge. It is as under: There are *two most frequent modes* of treatment to restore the ability of thyroid to produce hormones.

The first one is by use of strong dose of radioactive iodine to destroy cells in the thyroid gland. Radioactive iodine makes a trial to halt excess hormone production by thinning the ranks of cells responsible for producing the hormones. It is the estimated size of the thyroid gland, which decides the amount of radioactive iodine to be taken. The size of thyroid gland is estimated by physical examination and by ultrasound. The result of the symptoms produced by the body after intake of radioactive iodine actually decides the amount to be given later. It is opined that the intake of radioactive iodine does not destroy or harm the surrounding tissues or organs of the thyroid gland. The radioactive iodine is in the form of capsule or liquid, which contains the radioactive iodine. There are no side effects known. The iodine enters the system and gets collected in the thyroid. The excess of it will be excreted out through urine. *When radioactive iodine is taken, it is better to drink more of water per day for a week so that excessive iodine is flushed out.* It is also advised by the doctors not to be in close contact with infants, children and pregnant women for a week after ingest of iodine. Normally, there are no complications excepts in some cases. There is inflammation or soreness in thyroid gland for which the doctors give aspirin or ibuprofen for relief. In most of the cases, the radioactive iodine is sufficient to correct the thyroid gland but if the condition does not improve for three months, another dose of iodine is given. Routine monthly checks of thyroid are however necessary during these three months.

The doctor keeps one thing in mind that radioactive treatment is not given to pregnant women because this chemical may destroy the fetus.

STEPS OF TREATMENT

1. When hyperthyroidism has been diagnosed and the symptoms are indicative of a mild disease, the doctor may put the patient on beta-blockers. Beta-blockers are drugs like *atenolol and propranolol*, which are generally used to treat heart diseases and high blood pressure. These are used to regularize the heartbeat and to remove the symptoms of worry and anxiety because of excess of adrenalin in the blood. If the thyroid is overactive, the symptoms may be palpitation, sweat and nervousness among other. It is for this condition that beta-blockers are prescribed. The doctor would like to know whether the patient is asthmatic or has any kind of heart disease before prescribing beta-blockers.

2. If the disease is not of mild nature, the patient may be given both antithyroid drugs and beta-blockers. *Antithyroid drugs like propylthiouracil and methimazole* are given to interfere with thyroid hormone production.

3. If the symptoms are improved by this therapy, the drugs may be stopped but a watch is kept for possible relapse. On a relapse, the drugs will continue and radioactive iodine or even surgery may be required.

4. Radioactive iodine therapy and antithyroid drugs are normally useful in slowing down thyroid hormone output but in case of developing the disorder before or during pregnancy and

the patient is reluctant to undergo iodine therapy or antithyroid drugs due to allergy to these drugs, the alternative is recommending the subtotal thyroidectomy.

5. If the symptoms have not improved by the above therapy, it will have to be seen whether the patient has a large goiter and if so, surgery is the alternative.

6. In case of no enlargement of goiter, the way out is probably radioactive iodine treatment.

7. In most of the cases, the side effects of the above medicines *(carbimazol)* are not there but it is always better to know that these medicines may produce some symptoms like nausea, skin rashes and hair loss. In such case, the doctor has to be informed. Very rarely, say one in a thousand may have *agranulocytosis* in which the number of white blood-cells decrease. In such a case, there will be high fever, stomatitis and sore throat or could be bronchopneumonia. The condition should be reported to the doctor.

8. The remedies as above, thought to be conventional in treatment, limit the thyroid's ability to manufacture thyroid hormone and they increase the chances that the patient may *develop hypothyroidism,* which is a serious condition marked by insufficient thyroid hormone production. To avoid such type of transition, it is always wise to be in touch with the doctor.

9. Eye problems occur in only about five percent of people with Grave's disease and those who get it need professional treatment. It is also seen that eye protrusion can continue even after the thyroid hormone levels are brought under control by treatment. It is also observed that almost half of those who develop exophthalmos will have mild protrusion that can be helped with simple treatment.

10. Those who get eye problems with Grave's disease do find temporary relief from the inflammation, redness, swelling or

pain through proper medication such as *predinisolone, methylpredinisolone or dexamethasone* as per the advice of the doctor. It is also improper to use these medicines for longer period of time as these medicines can lead to bone loss, muscle weakness and weight gain. Vision problems and complicated cases of eye protrusion can be corrected through radiation therapy and surgery. The help of the eye specialist should be taken for eye treatment.

HOMOEOPATHIC TREATMENT FOR HYPERTHYROIDISM

In treating hyperthyroidism, one factor should be kept in mind that the aim of the doctor should be to ascertain the involvement of the organs and tissues of the body besides thyroid. It has to be seen whether the nervous centers, the pancreas and the mucous membrane are also involved or not. The symptoms of the body are always to be kept in mind as in the case of other diseases. We come to the remedies first, which are generally used in the disease.

Belladonna atropa

As a matter of rule, this remedy acts best on three main systems, the heart and circulation, nerves and the brain, and the eyes. The thyroid is very rarely affected. The patient of *Bell.* is easily excitable and worried over trifles. He or she is emotional rather violent in emotions, the pulse is full, rapid and bounding. There is throbbing in the carotids and the body temperature in on the higher side but the skin may be dry or moist. The eyeballs are prominent and there is deep pain in the eyeballs. The pupils are dilated, the mucous membrane is dry and the lids are stiff, swollen and dry. Tremors are also existing in some patients. The patient is full blooded and there is tendency of high blood pressure.

- The patient is plethoric, vigorous individual and intellectual.

- The patient narrates his or her symptoms complaining of violent heat, an unusual way to start with. Burning and redness is also reported. In some cases, the head is hot and the feet are cold or head is hot and both feet and hands are cold.
- There is great heaviness of the head. The head feels heavy and is drawn back from contraction of the muscles of the neck when the membranes of the upper portion of the spine are involved.
- The patient has great dryness, a sensation of dryness. There is dryness in the nose, mouth, tongue, throat, and chest for which the evidence is dry cough and spasmodic condition.
- The patient has an irritable state of mind affecting the urinary tract. There is irritation in the bladder with urging to urinate constantly. Either the urine dribbles or stops but this is due to some brain troubles.
- The complaints are right sided and most of them are acute conditions with thyroid problems.
- The patient is sleepy but cannot sleep. There is sweat on covered parts. If it is a child, grinding of teeth during sleep is there and the patient will cry in sleep suddenly but cry will cease suddenly as if nothing had been the matter.
- The patient's symptoms are aggravated from exposure to draft of air especially when the affected part is head. He or she wants to be wrapped up, the least jarring even light and noise aggravates suffering. Even talking creates a concussion in the sore parts and there is aggravation from lying down. The amelioration is from bending the affected parts backwards and inwards and also from warmth.

Ferrum phosphoricum

This remedy should be considered basically for anaemic patients for extremely nervous type. There is flushing of face when the patient is least excited unlike dark red of Gelsemium. After the flush is gone and excitement is over the face turns pale while the lips and mouth get paler than the face. 'Heart hurry' is the ranking symptom of this group for this remedy. The pulse is rapid, full and yet soft. While describing *Ferr.*, Boericke says that heart suddenly bleeds itself into the blood vessels and suddenly draws a reflex, leaving pallor of surface. But this is also true for *Ferr.* Eyelids are felt as if dry and as if there is sand under the lids. In women, the menses are too frequent and too profuse and some are reported to have bright red epistaxis.

Ferr-p. has little action on thyroid as we have said about Bell. but more important are the accompanying symptoms. Here it is eyes, which have plenty of symptoms. Besides that, it has more than plenty of symptoms on heart.

- The patient is not full-blooded and robust but nervous, sensitive, anaemic with false plethora and easy flushing.
- The patient corresponds to Grauvogl's oxygenoid constitution, the inflammatory, febrile, emaciating and wasting consumptive. (Boericke)
- There is aversion to milk and meat and desire for stimulants, sour eructation and vomiting of undigested food.
- The diurnal enuresis occurs and urine spurts with every cough. (Check with *Causticum* also)
- The neck is stiff with rheumatic pain in the shoulders. It can be used in the first stage of all inflammatory affections.
- The patient is worse at night, early morning (say from 4 to 6 a.m.), by touch, jar, motion and lying on the right side and feels better by cold applications.

Iodium

There is an opinion of some doctors that *Iodium* is of not much use for hyperthyroidism and its continuous use may aggravate the condition. But there are many doctors, who recommend that proper use and proper preparation of iodine does wonders in this disease. It should be used in 3rd potency, about 5 drops four times daily. These doctors state that there is no other remedy, which has so marked an affinity and so profound an effect on the glands as iodine and its compounds have.

To study this aspect, we have to keep in mind that thyroid gland has some amount of iodine or the nature of drug found in the thyroid resembles form of iodine existing in sea water. Any resemblance to iodine means that affections can be cured by the similar remedy, iodine and in case of aggravations found in use of iodine in some patients may be due to excessive use or improper use of iodine orally. We have discussed about *Ferr-p.* and *Bell.* above and find that there is some resemblance between *Ferr-p.* and *Bell.* and *Iod. Iod.* is more near to *Ferr-p* than *Bell.* In both the remedies, the patient is anemic and plethoric.

The basic difference between the three remedies that while *Ferr-p.* and *Bell.* do not act directly on thyroid gland, *Iod.* acts on thyroid, eyes, heart and nerves.

- There is goiter with a sensation of constriction and swollen submaxillary glands.
- Thyroid gland is enlarged and larynx feels constricted. There is pain in larynx and inspiration is difficult and the heart action is violent.
- There is palpitation from least exertion.
- There are flushes of heat all over the body with profuse attacks of sweating although the skin is dry.

Spongia tosta

Compare this remedy with *Iod.* and you will find a striking difference. The difference is that in *Iod.*, the patient is dark haired with dark yellow and tawny skin. He or she is restless and easily excitable. In *Spong.*, we have light hair, fair complexion and lax figured patient. Mental excitement aggravates all the subjective symptoms of *Spong.*, especially when they belong to hyperthyroid sufferings. The objective symptoms are constriction of larynx, pressure on larynx, sensation of dryness, and heat. A feeling as if a plug in the larynx has been fixed is also there.

- The patient is awakened suddenly after midnight with pain and suffocation.
- There is surging of heart into the chest as if it would force out upwards.
- The patient cannot lie down and has violent palpitations with dyspnea.
- There is itching, swelling and induration of glands.
- There is exhaustion and heaviness of the body after slight exertion with orgasm of blood to the chest and face. Anxiety and difficult breathing.
- The patient is worse before midnight, during winds and ascending; feel better while desending and lying with head low.
- The patient may have dry, barking cough with sounds of crowing or sawing. No rattling. The sound of breathing coming from the chest is like a saw driven through a pine tree.

Lycopus virginicus

Lycps-v. is basically a heart remedy, which reduces the rate of the heart and increases the length of systole to a great degree. In exophthalmic goiter, it is well indicated provided the other symptoms of the body relate to the remedy.

Under the heart, the symptoms will be that heart's action tumultuous and forcible; pulse weak, irregular, intermitent, tremulos, rapid, palpitation from nervous irritation with constriction and oppression in the precordial region. Eyes feel pushed out, with tumultuous action of the heart, is another prominent symptom. *Lycps-v.* is called the 'stock' remedy for the homoeopaths.

Pilocarpus microphyllus (Jaborandi)

Pilocarpus microphyllus is a powerful remedy for glandular stimulation and is most efficient diaphoretic. It directly acts upon the thyroid and its soporific action may possibly be due to abnormal sweats and night sweats. It is useful in exophthalmic goiter, with increased heart's action and pulsation of arteries; tremors and nervousness; heat and sweating; bronchial irritation. There is eye strain from whatever cause. Pupils are contracted and do not react to light. There is smarting pain in the eyes with white spots before the eyes.

Excessive perspiration from all parts of the body is a leading symptom of the remedy. The sweating is in paroxysms.

VIEWS OF GEORGE ROYAL

In his introductory explanation of this disease, Royal quotes *W.H. Dickinson*:

"A peculiar disease combining three characteristic conditions, namely: protrusion of eyeballs, enlargement of the thyroid gland and functional disturbance of the heart, chiefly manifested in accelerated heart beat symptoms, have been added by two others, viz., muscular tremors and elevated temperature of the skin with profuse heat and palpitations."

The disease is more frequent in males but more dangerous in women; violent emotions (fear, anger and grief) were given as the exciting causes. Acting through the sympathetic nerves upon the patient of a highly excitable, hysterical temperament and a constitution, weakened by loss of blood, prolonged lactation or diarrhea, or excessive mental work, are predisposing causes. This was all quoted fifty years ago when Royal wrote (1923).

[George Royal, W.H. Dickinson and J.M. Anders were professors in the State University of Iowa, college of Homoeopathic medicine.]

To the above symptoms, Anders added the influence of heredity, traumatism, physical strain and mental over work, toxemias and last and most important dysfunction of the internal glands, especially the adrenals. I say most important because this fact helps to establish for the location and the elective affinity of our remedies.

We have already given the four pathognomonic symptoms, viz., tremors, which are involuntary and fine, may number from 425 to 500 per minute.

Palpitation of the heart that accompanies the tachycardia is at first light but rapidly increases, usually brought on, and always aggravated by any mental excitement. The heartbeats run from 100 to 160. I had one case cured by *Ferr-p*. 30th, in which under the excitement heart beat often reached 180. The leading, and sometimes all the symptoms of neurasthenia may be present. Great excitability, mental depression and melancholia are frequent symptoms. In rare cases, which rapidly terminate fatally we may have mania. The exophthalmos varies in different patients and also in the same patient at different times. Immobility of the upper lid, a line of the white color noticeable above and below the cornea, and marked dryness of the membrane, are three important symptoms. Slight temporary retraction of the upper lid occurs if the eyes are fixed and an object is moved rapidly before them. Abnormalities of the optic nerve are rare, ulcers of the cornea may also occasionally occur. The arteries of the retina may pulsate with the heart beat. The pupils and the vision undergo no changes. The skin symptoms are slight rise of temperature, sometimes profuse sweating urticaria and pruritus, in advance cases edema, especially of the ankles, and inability to wrinkling of skin of the forehead. Some have also noted a marked decrease in the resistance to the electric current. Frequent flushing of the face, epistaxis, vomiting and purging, albuminuria, are the symptoms met in the disease.

The *diagnosis* is easy in the early stages, it may be mistaken for functional diseases of the heart but the appearance of the other three pathognomonic symptoms will soon settle the diagnosis.

Prognosis: The patient may continue in fair condition of health for many years as the disease is essentially a chronic one. Complete restoration of the patients to health is rare. Some cases terminate fatally in a short time in spite of all treatment. It is generally conceded that the best surgeons now and then, either remove or injure the parathyroid glands and cause death, from tetany, in a few days.

The treatment should be medical (drug), surgical and auxiliary, according to the etiology as it is understood today. The surgical treatment has been too much emphasized. It is useless to remove a part or the entire thyroid gland of the patient when the cause of hyperthyroidism is in one of the internal glands, in one or more septic foci, or in the occupation or environment of the patient, if these exciting causes are not removed by the operation. We should employ our drug therapy and auxiliary treatment before and after operating. In other words, surgery should be the last resort.

REPERTORY SUGGESTIONS

Pain, thyroid gland: Am-c., Carb-v., Cupr., Spig.

Pain, thyroid gland, moving head on: Iod.

Pain, thyroid, right: Alum., Caust., Merc-i-f., Vesp.

Pain, thyroid, left: Berb., Coloc., Form., Nat-s.

Pain, thyroid, pressing: Bar-c.

Paint, thyroid, soreness: Ail., Kali-i., Nicc.

Pain, thyroid, stitching: Am-c., Iod., Nat-c., Spong., Sulph.

Pain, thyroid, swallowing: Spong.

Swelling, thyroid gland: Ail., Ars., Aur-s., Carb-an., Caust., Clem., Kali-i., Nat-c., Nit-ac., Ol-j., Thuj.

Swelling, thyroid gland, right: Merc.

Swelling, thyroid gland, right sensation of: Mag-c.

Swelling, thyroid, veins: Hyos., Nat-m., Op., Stry., Thuj.

Tension, thyroid gland: Agar.

Tickling, thyroid gland: Kali-c.

Tingling, thyroid gland: Calc.

COMMON REMEDIES

Bell., Bufo, Ferr-p., Iod., Lycps-v., Nat-m.

With trembling: Meph.

With cardiac symptoms: Cact.

With choking sensation: Graph., spong.

Painful, during menses: Iod.

Rapid heart action: Bufo.

Lumpy appearance: Graph.

Hard: Bufo, Iod., Nat-c., Spong.

Nodulated: Graph., Phyt.

With palpitations: Phos.

Pains during pregnancy: Calc-i., Hydr.

Vascular: Apis, Calc.

GENERAL

Eats well but loses weight: Iod.

Eats well but loses weight, worse after shock or grief: Nat-m.

Constitutional medicines are the best to use and the consideration is to be given for *Calc., Lach., Puls.* and *Graph.* Select one and then give *Thyr.* 200 or 1M as intermediate remedy.

Calc-f. 6x and *Calc-p.* 6x can be given in biochemic remedies along with selected constitutional remedy.

Therapeutic Suggestions

LET THERE be any name of the disease related to endocrine glands, one aspect is clear that some of the remedies are particularly meant for endocrine disorders. It remains to be studied in a comparative way to find out the therapeutic value of each. Here is an attempt.

CRETINISM

In our practice, we find little patients having dull and backward mind and body. They generally respond quite well to the *Calcarea* group of remedies, *Silicea* and *Sulphur*. Besides these remedies, *Natriums* and *Kalis* are also taken into account and proved successful when indicated. The most useful remedies for such children are those which are constitutional. It takes time to find out which one is the constitutional for a particular child but once it is found and applied, one can see the wonders of homoeopathy. The underdeveloped, dull, stupid, slow-learning and nervous children fed with constitutional remedies resort to normal development within years. If such children are deceitful in their behaviour along with their backwardness and also get convulsions, one can think of remedies like *Argentum nitricum* and *Bufo rana*.

According to *Robert*, consideration of the mental and emotional states is best indication for the simillimum. This is not as simple as to feed glandular preparations, perhaps, but it is less apt to throw other glandular secretions out of proportion, and the results seem to be generally better. And no man who has watched the action of our potencies can doubt the efficacy of the medicines.

GOITER, HYPERTHYROID AND HYPOTHYROID

To a great extent the remedies, which come to mind as constitutional remedies of sufficient depth to influence these glandular conditions with their structural and nervous concomitants, are *our great polychrests,* and many of these are from the same chemical base as the elements of the physical body—*Sulphur, Silicea, Phosphorus, Kalis, Natriums,* and the *Carbons.* Then we find such remedies as *Lycopodium, Nitric acid,* and the major *nosodes,* of great use in these conditions.

RESCUE LEADER—SULPHUR

When we talk of polychrests, we cannot forget the greatest of all polychrests *Sulphur.* There is not a single organ in the body, which is not influenced by *Sulphur.* There is not a single function of the body, which is not impressed by this great polychrest. So far as glandular system is concerned, *Sulphur* has a lot to contribute and make influence on the glandular system. *Hering* has done a lot of work to prove *Sulphur* on the glandular system. In backward children, *Sulphur* is valuable. It is very much meaningful in deep rooted affections, which arise from the suppression of superficial symptoms. The dual action of *Sulphur* is well known to all. Not only that it can be given as per the symptoms but it can be used to stir the organism to react when the seemingly indicated remedies fail to act, especially if there are recurrences of acute or sub-acute manifestations, where the patient moves toward recovery only to slip back repeatedly.

HELPER—PHOSPHORUS

Next to *Sulphur* is *Phosphorus.* It has a different lay out than *Sulphur* because of its classical constitution not resembling any other medicine. Where *Sulphur* is indolent (lazy), *Phosphorus* is excitable, rather over excitable and erotic in many diseases. It has erratic sexual symptoms like impotence, lascivious ideas, and insanity to any extent- so far as sex is concerned, vicarious menstruation and abnormal labors. All these are somewhat related to glandular dysfunctions. *Phosphorus* also affects the development of the physical body in the child and also makes a difference in the mental activity so far as concentration in studies, etc. is concerned. It is true for *Sulphur* too but with a difference in constitution. Prostrated energies from loss of fluids and from emotional and physical strains point towards *Phosphours*, as against the general lack of energy in *Sulphur*.

BROTHER—ACID PHOSPHORICUM

Next to *Phosphorus* is its brother *Acid phosphoricum*. This should not be forgotten while undertaking glandular difficulties and glycosuria.

SMOOTHING EDGE—LACHESIS

The most frequent imbalance of functioning of endocrine glands occurs in women when they approach menopause. Although thyroid problems mostly attack women before they achieve menopause but exceptions are there when thyroid problems also start along. Such patients have ample of well-marked subjective symptoms, which mostly lead to *Lachesis*.

QUEEN OF CURE—PULSATILLA

While checking with suitable rubrics for glandular conditions concerning thyroid, we cannot forget the credit of *Pulsatilla*. *Pulsatila* is not conspicuous or prominent in curing thyroid disease because many of its rubrics are missing. Even if they are found, they are in a lower rating. It is basically a woman remedy having emotional background too and there is every likelihood of misusing this remedy by the homoeopaths. If *Pulsatilla* comes in mind, think of *Lycopodium* first. According to *Hering, Lycopodium* is one of the very few survivors from the first era of plant life, and it has changed very little in appearance. It has survived because of the basic qualities inherent in the development of all life, and probably, therefore, has a greater potential influence on organic functions.

SENSITIVE MATE—*NITRICUM ACIDUM*

When we talk of glandular dysfunctions, there is no reason why *Nitricum acidcum* should not be considered in the discussions? In case there are certain symptoms indicating that the patient's disease is of syphilitic origin, *Nit-ac.* comes in the first row. *We have already discussed in the miasms chapter that Nit-ac. is antipsoric and antisycotic.* The keynote of this remedy is sensitiveness. Sensitiveness of the affected parts, head, to touch, jars, sudden motions, sudden change in tempo of motion, to cold, to change in weather, tendency to take cold and so on. There is great disturbance of the circulation of blood in the fingers and toes. They appear livid, pale cold or dead at times. There is a sensation of a splinter in the throat, and tonsils. So far as sexual trend is concerned, in *Nit- ac.*, the disturbance of sexual organs and functions rivals *Phosphorus*, and sometimes there is almost as much lasciviousness.

MAGICAL TRIO—*SULPHUR, CALCAREA CARBONICA* AND *LYCOPODIUM*

We come the great trio of Clarke, *Sulph, Calc. and Lyc.* These are wonderful remedies for acute glandular affections. *Clarke says*, "All the rest of materia medica can be grouped" and they will not offer such brilliant results as shown by this trio. "This trio has swollen glands, and is one of the few specifically mentioned as having *goiter*" says *Roberts*.

From among this trio, *Lyc.* is one of the few remedies mentioned in the materia medica as definitely rending to enlargement of bony tissue. If you check with *Phos.*, it has no enlargement but thickness of bony tissue. *Lyc.* has a furrowed face and forehead, thin face, neck and upper chest while the remaining body below chest goes plump. There is progressive emaciation from above downwards. Tiredness, weariness, lassitude, pain in legs while taking rest in the night or after slight exertion and want of bodily heat are some of the symptoms relating to the glandular diseases. In *Lyc.*, the fingers feel numb and dead as in *Nit-ac.* Mentally, *Lyc.*, is as fearful as *Phos.* and the *Kalis*, as sad as *Nit-ac.* and the *Natriums*. While we talk of burning, we are reminded that burning pains of *Lyc.* make us think of *Sulph.* and *Phos.*

THE CHRONIC GROUP HEALER—*NATRIUM MURIATICUM*

We now come to *Natrium* group of remedies. *Natrium* represents the mental depression and general state of gloominess (melancholy) especially in chronic diseases. *Natriums* are averse to consolation and have changing mood from gloominess to gaiety and vice-versa. Besides mental action, the physical side involves chemistry of fluids in the body and also pathology of the organs. *Natriums* bring sudden feeling of weakness, sudden failing of strength, sudden exhaustion of sexual organs due to excessive stimulation, sudden and rapid changes in the blood, sudden and profound emaciation, and excessive drainage of the body fluids coming on suddenly.

Leading among *Natriums* is *Natrium muriaticum* which has direct link to the neck glands (thyroid). It reduces the size of neck i.e. profound emaciation about the neck even when the patient eats ravenously. *The group of remedies affects the thyroid gland markedly and has the subjective sensation of compression, as if there were a lump or plug in the throat* Take the instance of *Natrium arsenicosum*, It has a sensation as if the thyroid body were compressed between the thumb and finger. Check with *Natrium carbonicum*. Now, it has the hard swelling of thyroid. Again take *Nat-m*. It is full of tears. Tears with emotional depression, tears with laughter and seeing comic scenes on TV, seeing tragic ends on TV shows bring tears, tears with onset of coryza and tears with cough. The strong desire for salt is more marked in *Nat-m*. Glandular imbalance or thyroidism in any shape can be connected with this salt provided the patient had a history of malaria and taken doses of quinine. We have talked of *Ign.* in our therapeutics for goiter. *Nat-m.* is supposed to be chronic of *Ign*. Hence, the emotional *Natriums* show the effects of emotional strain or shock as much as that of *Ignatia*.

WHITE SPLENDOR OF *KALIUMS*

The patients of *Kali* family are generally short in stature, chubby to obese in shape and classical sycotic, having anaemia. This is a perfect picture of *Kali* tallying with characteristic mental symptoms, which exhibit an imbalance in endocrine system. There is loss of memory, dull mentality and helplessness to exert more of brains in any affair, easily startled at the slightest noise, fearful, apprehensive and predict their death. *Kali* is as sad as *Natrium but Kali* is more fearful. Mental exertion aggravates the symptoms of Natriums but Kalis cannot concentrate enough to bring an aggravation.

Kalium arsenicum is very useful in exophthalmic goiter. In backward children with cretinism *Kalium bromatum* and *Kalium phosphoricum* have done good work. Marked anaemia, pale young people who flush easily, disturbed menstrual function, atrophy of male organs and nervous people suffering from insomnia are good symptoms for *Kali-p.*, especially when glandular disease associates these symptoms.

Kali iod. is one of our great remedies for goiter. Besides it has atrophy of mammae and testes. Life appears insupportable to Kali-

i. and the patient awakens at night with dread of sleep further till dawn.

Kali mur. is the wonderful member of Kali family, which has swollen glands, be it *goiter*, thyroid, even swelling following cuts, bruises. It is very helpful in glandular problems following vaccination and in Hodgkin's disease.

THE WONDERFUL EARTHY—*SILICEA*

Silicea has an important relationship to growth, development and functions of the mind and body. A brief mention is here made in appreciation of using *Sil.* in thyroid diseases when there is suppression of foot sweat and vaccination as the cause of problems. In cretinism, the use of *Silicea* and *Calcarea* group medicines can be taken. *Calcarea* can be considered in corpulent adults with full abdomen (pot bellied in children) and goiter or renal calculi.

There are other remedies belonging to carbons for glandular conditions. These are Carb-v., Carb-an., Graph., and Sep. These remedies can be used according to symptoms in all conditions of thyroid disease. As a matter of rule, all the polychrests are bound to yield good results in endocrine disorders.

I end this topic here with a wonderful quote from Herbert A. Roberts on endocrine disorders.

"As homoeopathic physicians, we have undertaken a labor that is vast in its expanse, yet it yields to us in the degree to which we apply ourselves in its pursuit. Our resources are far greater than those of the orthodox school; we have proved them to be potent in a varying range of attenuations to suit the best to each man's experience and requirements. Our remedies will not upset the *balance of endocrine secretions*, for the simillimum will fill the demands of the system in all its parts without stimulating too much those organs which have maintained a relatively secure balance. In other words, our remedies affect directly the vital energy, which in itself establishes equilibrium, those parts which are susceptible because of the imbalance becoming a part of normal healthy functioning of the whole unit. Let us watch with great interest the investigation of the endocrine system, but let us look with the expectant eye of the explorer upon our homoeopathic remedies, that we may meet and cure even these little-understood conditions."

■

Differential Diagnosis of Swelling of the Neck

SIDE OF THE NECK

Swelling in the side of the neck is very common and is due to enlargement of the deep cervical lymph nodes. There may be enlarged submandibular salivary gland with the lymph nodes in the submandibular triangle. This may also extend from the jaws. In the carotid triangle, carotid body tumor, branchial cyst and bronchogenic carcinoma may also exist. Thyroid swelling will lie deep to the sternomastoid. In the posterior triangle, there may be cystic hygroma or a lipoma besides the lymph nodes.

There are two types of swelling on the side of neck, *acute swelling* and *chronic swelling*. *Acute* swelling is cellulitis including Ludwig's angina, boil, carbuncle and acute lymphadenitis. *Chronic* swelling may be *cystic, solid and pulsatile*.

In *cysts*, one may find branchial cyst, thyroglossal cyst, cystic hygroma, dermoid cyst, sebaceous cyst, tuberculous abscess and cystic adenoma of thyroid gland.

In *solid*, there is swelling due to the lymph nodes, submandibular salivary gland, thyroid gland and cervical rib.

In *pulsatile*, aneurysm of the carotid or subclanian artery and exophthalmic goiter are the indications.

MIDDLE SWELLINGS

Swelling in the middle of neck is from above downwards and it may be due to Ludwig's angina, enlarged submental lymph nodes, sublingual dermoid and lipoma in the submental region. Goiter of the thyroid isthmus and dermoid cyst may also be the reasons besides carcinoma of the larynx and cystic hygroma.

CELLULITIS

It comes up beneath the deep cervical fascia and it is the most serious form of cellulitis of the neck. The inflammatory exudates are held tightly under tension by the unyielding deep fascia and tend to tract towards the mediastinum. In such a case, the neck is very painful and stiff. On palpation, an indurated feel is obtained. We have earlier talked of *Ludwig's angina*. For information, it is stated that it is a form of cellulitis that starts in the submandibular region and spreads to the floor of the mouth. It brings a diffuse swelling below the jaw, often fixing the tongue. As a result of this sort of swelling, there may be serious complications like edema glottis, mediastinitis and fatal septicemia during the course of cellulitis.

BRANCHIAL CYST

Branchial cyst is mostly found in the adults and adolescents, although one of the factors for this type of swelling is congenital. The swelling is mostly of an oval shape and it is deep to the upper third of the sternomastoid, divided half way in the front and behind the muscle. The diagnosis may be ascertained by finding cholesterol crystals in the aspirated fluid.

CARBUNCLE

Carbuncle produces a type of diffuse brawny indurated swelling mostly in the back of neck.

DIFFERENTIAL DIAGNOSIS OF THYROID SWELLING

When the patient of thyroid comes to the homoeopath, it becomes essential to fit him or her in some frame of disease before the symptomatic study, according to rule, is done.

A thyroid swelling has to be examined first by its situation or position, size and shape of swelling and by the observation that the swelling moves up and down when the patient is told to conduct the act of swallowing.

ACUTE THYROIDITIS

When the patient has suffered from some enteric or infective fever and comes to the doctor with a swelling in the neck, thyroid gland will be hot and tender. Such cases of acute thyroidits are rare.

RIEDLE'S THYROIDITIS OR STRUMA FIBROSA

In this disorder, the thyroid gland becomes stony hard due to progressive increasing sclerosis of the thyroid gland. The sclerosis process may extend beyond the thyroid gland and then it involves the sheath, trachea and esophagus.

HASHIMOTO'S DISEASE

It generally affects the women who are under the process of achieving menopause or have just passed the menopause. In this case, the thyroid gland is enlarged and has well defined margin with rubber like consistency. In the case of Hashimoto's disease the physician should check the spleen and liver. These are found enlarged in some cases.

LYMPHADENOID GOITER

This disease affects the small girl most. In it, the inflammatory process is as found in Riedel.

GOITER

All non-inflammatory and non-neoplastic swellings of the thyroid gland are called goiter. Goiter is classified into *simple* and *toxic* categories. In simple goiter, there are three varieties, *parenchymatous, diffuse colloid* and *nodular* whereas in toxic goiter, there are two categories, *primary* and *secondary*. Let us take them one by one.

Parenchymatous goiter

Children and adolescents between the age of 5 to 20 years are affected by this type of goiter in the endemic areas. It has to be noted that some physiological hyperplasia occurs in the girls at puberty and in women during pregnancy and also at the time of menopause. This type of goiter subsides on its own or with the help of iodine therapy. If this does not happen due to normal involution, it may subsequently end in a diffuse colloid or nodular goiter.

Diffuse colloid goiter

As stated above, the thyroid in such case becomes enlarged, soft and elastic. No other difficulty is indicated and pressure application over it is also rare unless the swelling is more.

Nodular goiter

In this variety of goiter, two conditions are noted. They may be either single or multiple or we can say that they are solitary nodular goiter or multinodular goiter. The solitary nodular goiter is usually sporadic and the multinodular goiter is endemic. The solitary nodule may be present any where in the thyroid gland and its site is junction of isthmus and one lateral lobe.

The patient experiences dyspnoea and disfigurement initially. Toxic symptoms appear later. Complications like hemorrhage, calcification, secondary toxicosis and carcinoma may develop in the nodular type. Sudden hemorrhage into the goiter is the reason for dyspnoea and this condition may need tracheotomy.

Grave's disease or exophthalmic goiter

This term can be called *primary toxic goiter* also and this happens in healthy gland. There is a history of strains, worry, overwork, and severe mental depression in the patients suffering from Grave's disease. In most of the cases of Grave's disease there are four characteristics, *exophthalmos, and enlargement of thyroid gland, tachycardia and tremor*. Further there may be loss of weight, more of thirst, and irregular menstrual function, usually amenorrhoea. The BMR or basal metabolic rate is as high as 100 percent.

Secondary toxic goiter

There is a toxicity noted on the previously diseased gland just opposite to primary toxic goiter, which has a previous healthy history of the gland. The previous history is mostly a nodular goiter. Actually the attack of disease is on cardiovascular system. There may be no exophthalmos, no tremors and no tachycardia but on the other hand, the pulse becomes irregular in rate and rhythm. The patient feels precordial exhaustion and pain, which in due course or later forms into auricular fibrillation and heart failure.

Retrosternal goiter

In this type of goiter, there is no swelling of the thyroid or any swelling observed on the neck. When the patient sleeps on one side, say right or left, he or she feels dysponeic. The evident and most diagnostic feature is the presence of engorged veins over the upper part of the chest. This can be easily confirmed by taking X-ray pictures.

Tumors

Benign tumors are very rare and the eventuality is mostly *carcinoma*, which is of two types, the *papillary*, occurring in the young and the *nonpapillary*, occurring in the old. The diagnosis is by the hard feel and indistinct outline of the thyroid swelling. Gradually, it infiltrates into the neighbouring structures like the trachea, esophagus recurrent laryngeal nerve, infrahyoid muscles etc. Thereby causing dyspnoea, dysphagia and hoarseness of voice. On the other hand, the carotid sheath is surrounded by the growth so that its pulsation cannot be felt at the back of swelling.

Thyroglossal Cyst

It is situated in the midline or just lateral to it. It moves upwards when the tongue is protruded, besides that, it moves up and down when in the act of swallowing.

SECTION - 2

Alternative Therapies

THE MODERN era has reached a stage where all rational ideas get a thinking if not implementation. Recently, alternative therapies have found a good seat in the treatment of diseases. Some people think that Homoeopathy is also an alternative therapy to which I do not agree. Homoeopathy has now achieved a different and recognizable status not only in public but in the government circles as well. Its reputation in India is much more if compared with other countries. Some people call Homoeopathy as a complementary therapy, which is also natural. It is not complementary but a separate distinguished branch of medicine-system that has been fully proved and authenticated by the tools of science. Dealing with acute diseases has been the property of the orthodox system of medicines because of its efficacy of suppression and healing. Acute diseases are of those nature, which can be identified, diagnosed and then treated. Serious and chronic illnesses like tuberculosis and other infectious diseases including thyroid diseases take long time to get cured. They are not well cured by orthodox system of medicines and in some cases (thyroid diseases is one of them), the medicines are to be taken throughout the life. Thyroid diseases take several years to get cured fully. In the mean time, when the medicines of orthodox system are continued to be taken by the patient, there is no harm if alternative ways are adopted for preventing symptoms to get alleviated or prevented from progressing. Good healers or doctors never object to such a therapy that is not going to harm the patient physically but going to improve them both mentally and physically. It is not the method of treatment but the mental satisfaction, which is going to cure the person. There are many alternative therapies like Yoga, Acupuncture, Acupressure, Reflexology, Massaging, and Reiki etc. Any one of them can be selected according to suitability, availability and choice. The results can be seen with one therapy after trying for at least three months and if you do not find any difference or benefit, you may switch over to the next alternative therapy. Yoga, will not let you down, if it is done under the guidance of a perfect master.

The best part of the alternative therapy is that while you get treatment from the orthodox system or the system of homoeopathic medicines, you are a passive recipient, whatever your doctor advises, you have to carry out in terms of medicines. In adopting alternative therapies, you may be asked to change your life style, your diet, and your habits and do some exercises. *Body when strengthened through alternative therapy will be commanding you to be fit. You become an active participant in your treatment.*

THE IMBALANCE AND THE ALTERNATIVE THERAPY

There is another aspect concerning alternative therapy. Alternative therapy is much related with the balancing act of your body. Thyroid disease is an act of imbalance. It is an imbalance connected with the hormones. This imbalance is supposed to be a caused due to illness and our body has the power to heal it by balancing the body and put it on a right path of healing. The medicines also perform the same act of balancing but the alternative therapy by its physical impact (through exercise) energizes the body. We can see it from another angle especially when we talk of Ayurveda, the ancient art of healing in India. In *ayurveda*, most of the medicines are from minerals and herbs. The ancient concept of 'cold' and 'hot' in ayurveda fits perfectly in the thyroid disease. Thyroid gland is the generator of the body and its function is mainly connected with the hot and cold, which fits directly into the theory of endocrinology of the modern era of medicines. If the body is cold and feels cold, the person is likely to have a sluggish metabolism and also has a tendency to get obese. On the other hand, if a person is hot and feels hot, he or she will have a high metabolic rate and find him/herself stressed and nervous. Leave aside ayurveda, consider *Acupuncture* or *Acupressure*, these therapies also believe in hot and cold phenomenon of the body thereby confirming that balance is key to cure. These theories balance the two opposite qualities, *Yin* and *Yang*. These theories are, therefore, successful in treating many hormonal based disorders.

AYURVEDA IN THYROID PROBLEMS

Coming to ayurveda, man is microcosm [world of man; man as epitome of universe] of nature. There are five elements present in all matters in each individual. These five elements have to be in balance if a perfect health is desired. Any imbalance can lead to diseases. These five elements are *Ether, Air, Fire, Water* and *Earth*. There are many spaces in the body, which are manifestations of the *Ether* element. Thorax, mouth, respiratory tract, gastrointestinal tract, tissues, cells, lymphatic and capillaries are the spaces in the body. *Air* is the second element, which is responsible for movements. The heart, the contraction and expansion of lungs and movement of intestines relate to air element. *Fire* is the source of metabolism in the body. It works in digestion, brain-cells, induces intelligence, perceives light through retina, controls body-temperature and gives power of thinking. *Water* is the fourth element in the body that secretes digestive juices, makes salivary glands work, besides that its manifestations activate mucous membranes, plasma and cytoplasm. Water is a vital element for functioning of tissues and other body systems. In case of dehydration due to some disease, the water in the body becomes water of life, if not recouped. *Earth is the fifth element of the body*. Without a base like earth, the body cannot remain stable on earth. It holds the body to the earth in the form of bones, cartilage, nails, muscles, skin, hair and tendons etc. So, the five elements as above form a body.

PITTA AND THYROID

From the above explanation, it is evident that each element holds a position in the body and that body cannot live without the harmonious help of each other. *Fire element is responsible for metabolism and it is this, which is connected with our thyroid.* Another element water is also connected with thyroid. We discussed about 'hot' and 'cold' condition of the body earlier while discussing about alternative therapy. So, both fire and water are actually important for the disease of thyroid. All these elements are based upon three main element *vata, pitta and kapha*. These govern all the biological, physiopathological and psychological functions of the body. *Water and fire belong to pitta element.* It is *pitta*, which is the leader in the body for functions like body heat, temperature, digestion, perception, hunger, understanding, thirst, intelligence, anger, hatred and jealousy. Whenever there is variation in pitta element in the constitution, the body expresses itself in the form of various diseases and one of them is thyroid disease. We must remember that each body is a combination of all the three elements with a predominant tendency towards one manifestion '*dosha*' (fault more). Ayurveda is based upon the theory of these three elements and cause of the disease is due to imbalance in these three elements.

A PROBABLE CONSTITUTION OF THYROID DISEASE PERSONS

Here I give a rough idea of those who may have thyroid disease or having this disease. It is the 'pitta' element, which is not in balance and hence there is a need to discuss about 'pitta' constitution. Persons with 'pitta' constitution are medium height, delicate and having slender body-built. Their complexion may be coppery, reddish or yellowish with soft and warm skin with less of wrinkles and tendency to have premature gray hair. They may have moles, warts, freckles and their muscles are moderate with bones not much prominent. They have strong metabolism, good digestion and good appetite when the 'pitta' is in perfect order. They consume good quantity of food and water with craving for sweets, have astringent taste and like cold drinks. Their urine comes in abundance and sweating is excessive. Their body temperature is slightly more and their extremities are generally warm. They do not have the capability to tolerate too much of heat and cannot do much hard work. They have very fair power of comprehension and are quite intelligent. They are ambitious people and command the members of their family in all ways.

FOOD AND THYROID

Any type of convalescene is the period for regenerating the body's healing power and restoring the weakened immune system. At his juncture, even the orthodox system of medicine does not divert from the nutritional food and care by a dietician. All the hospitals have appointed dieticians for indoor patients. A good and balanced diet is important and vital for the work of generation and repair of the body besides the medicines. Food should be nourishing, easy on the digestion and of the liking of the patient to some extent.

In the case of thyroid diseases, first of all non-vegetarian foods should be totally stopped. This is possible in India but in other countries, where non-vegetarian food cannot be avoided, care has to be taken that no red meat should be taken. Red meat is difficult to digest. Besides this prevention, all fried and fatty foods should also be avoided for the same reason of digestion.

Now please note that the above qualities belong to 'pitta' quality of people. *Pitta dosha* have many manifestations of disease but we are concerned about thyroid and hence all this explanation.

Avoid following foods

To decrease 'pitta dosha' or avoid thyroid disease, one should not take spicy foods, peanuts or peanut butter, bananas, garlic, tomatoes, cherries, green grapes, lemons, sour oranges, sour pineapple, sour plums, apricots and sour fruits. It is not advisable to eat spicy or pungent food or hot food during summer when 'Pitta' is supposed to be at the peak during the year. Pungent vegetables, carrots, beets, garlic, onions, hot peppers, radishes, spinach etc. are not advisable. Brown rice, eggs (yolk), pork and seafood, buttermilk, cheese, yogurt, almond and corn oils are not to be taken.

People suffering from thyroid diseases should not take incompatible foods together. These foods are milk and fish, meat and milk, curds and beef, pickles and milk. If taken in combination as above, they are likely to increase the thyroid disease. Besides that, these can give rise to many skin diseases.

Take these foods

The foods which should be taken for people suffering from thyroid gland diseases are sweet fruits like apples, coconut, figs, mango, dark grapes, melons, sweet oranges, sweet plums, and sweet pineapples. They can take unsalted butter, cottage cheese, ghee, milk, use coconut oil and sunflower oil, eggs (white), chicken, sweet and bitter vegetables, cabbage, cauliflower, green beans, lettuce, mushrooms, peas, potatoes, sprouts and green peppers, rice (white and basmati), and wheat.

These are food guidelines for the constitutions suffering from 'pitta' dosha and not necessarily from thyroid disease. There are different conditions and layout of thyroid disease and for proper guidance, an ayurveda expert can only brief the patient. This is a rough layout.

YOGA AND THYROID DISEASES

We can say with ease that ayurveda and yoga are different methods to keep one healthy in the alternative therapies but they are sister sciences. It is quite traditional and customary to study ayurveda before yoga is taken up for practical aspects. Ayurveda is the science of the body and to keep the body fit, its medicines are used. Yoga is a way to life and it tones up the whole system physically and uplifts spiritually.

To maintain good health, the spiritual science of yoga comes in. A brilliant medicine-scholar named 'Patanjali' introduced yoga to the Indian medical sciences in ancient India and it is very useful for maintaining good health and to attain longevity. *Patanjali* described eight limbs of yoga and yogic practices. These eight limbs are nervous system, cleansing, discipline, postures, concentration, contemplation, awakening of awareness and the state of perfect equilibrium. Yoga exercises, when conducted, are preventive as well as curative.

In another explanation, *Patanjali* enumerates eight pillars of yoga, which relates to the body and mind. *These are Yama, Niyamas, Asanas, Pranayama, Pratyahar, Dhaarna, Dhyan and Samadhi.* These relate to eternal spiritual restraints (*yama*), social or behavioural restraint (*Niyamas*), different postures of body (*Asanas*), control of life-breath (*Pranayama*), withdrawal of senses from objects of indulgences (*Pratyahar*), selection of spiritual objects of dwelling within (*Dhaarna*), concentration on that spiritual object (*Dhyaan*) and atonement with spiritual entity (*Samadhi*).

As regards the eight eternal spiritual restraints (Yamas), *Patanjali* says in *Yoga darshan* that there are five eternal spiritual truths, which should guide us. These are non-violence, truth, nonacquisition, self-control, and surrender of material possession. They are basic principles of our life eternally true in all climates, times and places. We shall not go into the details of yoga because our main subject is its relation with thyroid.

Life is full of tensions. Not a moment passes without anxiety of some kind or the other. All the decisions we take are fraught with some element of tension. It is stress, which disturbs the metabolism of the body. Metabolism has direct link with thyroid. Yoga cushions us against the effect of stress on our metabolism. Moreover, if our life is based upon the yoga principles like non-violence, truth, non-acquisitiveness, self-control and dispossession, we shall be free from tension and stress.

If we say that Yoga is nothing but conduction of asanas, it is not true. Yoga is a very wide term. It is a psychological and spiritual way to life.

The best part of the yoga is that it balances the neurohormones and metabolism besides improving the endocrine metabolism. This is what is needed in the treatment of thyroid diseases.

In yoga, a discipline is maintained and some postures are made. These postures of the body are fashioned in such a way that these open up and move energies that have accumulated or stagnated in the energy centers. If the energy is centered in one location and gets stagnated, many ills are created. The stagnation is released by conducting yoga and disease-producing toxins are released cleaning the physical and psychological disorders.

It is again ayurveda, which guides the type of yoga, one should conduct and this is done according to the ailment and constitution of the body. Since we are concerned about thyroid disease, which is related to '*Pitta*' constitution, it is indicative of certain postures, which are not to be performed by pitta constitutions. For example 'shirshasana' (the head-stand posture) should not be done by thyroid-disease people. If it is done, there may be some mental disorientation.

ALTERNATIVE THERAPIES

DIRECTIONS FOR CONDUCTING YOGASANAS

- Yogasanas should be preferably done under the guidance of a master.
- Conducting yogasanas will bring better results if done empty stomach early in the morning.
- These should be done after evacuation of stools and cleaning of teeth.
- Breathing should be through nose and not through mouth while conducting asanas.
- Asanas are to be done in milder way, not exerting the body because it is not a warming exercise. Do them slowly and patiently.
- They should be done on the floor after spreading a comfortable mat or soft blanket so that the energy generated by the body does not go into earth.
- Do not go out after the asanas when the climate is either very cold or hot. Wait for some time. The best place for conducting them is in a garden.
- There should be very less clothing on the body and the clothing should be loose and not tight to the body. In winters, one can have soft and loose woollens to avoid exposures.
- After conducting asanas, try to urinate.
- It is better to drink some quantity of fresh water after some time of the asanas.
- Pregnant women should not conduct asanas without the advise of a master.

YOGA-ASANAS BENEFICIAL FOR THYROID DISEASE

Before the postures are discussed, the first one that can be tried is the breathing exercise or 'Pranayama' This exercise is excellent in bringing back the faith and balance of the mind. There is a feeling of peace and tranquility, purity of mind and joyful bliss felt in the body and life after doing it. There are different types of 'Pranayamas' but for curing thyroid diseases, the one that suits is as follows:

Pranayama

Pranayama is the fourth part of the eight fold yoga described in the yogasutra of Patanjali. The initial manifestation of life in a newborn baby is to take a deep breath. This first breathing is called *Prana* because without it, the baby cannot survive. This ritual is without any training to the baby who takes breathing inside, retains it for a while and then releases the breathing. This is the process of breathing against which life commences. The life ends when this breathing ceases to exist. One can live without food or water for sometime but one cannot live without breathing. To attain good health, breathing has to be controlled and vitalized by some method of breathing in and breathing out. *Pranayama* is developed to look into this very aspect of breathing properly.

Our ancient books on health reveal that there are three steps in conducting *Pranayama*. Inhaling air into the lungs with all strength is the first step and is called *poorak*.

Holding back the air in the lungs is the second step called *kumbhaka*.

Final exhaling the air from lungs is the third step called *rechaka*.

Poorak should be for about 10 seconds, Kumbhak should be for about 40 seconds and rechak should be for 20 seconds (average for a healthy person). Actually this depends upon the capacity of the individual and is variable.

The pranayama suitable for thyroid disease is that you inhale through left nostril and exhale through right nostril, using thumb and middle finger to close and open alternate nostril by pressing the side of the nose. Do it for at least ten times. Now comes the second step. Inhale through left nostril and hold your breath for some time. Now release the breath i.e. exhale till the time you can do so and hold it for some time. This requires practice. The time to hold should be according to one's capacity to do so and in no case any longer time should be given beyond capacity. This exercise creates a cooling effect in the body and increases the energy especially in women. After this exercise for a few days, you will find yourself a new person free of depression and tension. *It is my sincere advice to the readers that yoga should not be done without proper training otherwise there may be some adverse effects.*

Neck movements

Forward and backward movement

There is a special need for making the neck more flexible which makes thyroid gland work properly. For this, neck movement is an essential need. The exercise is very simple and can be done while lying down on the bed. Place a lean pillow below the neck, not beneath the head. Now move the head forward and backward alternatively. If this exercise is done while standing, there will be more of fatigue. If no fatigue is felt, this can be done in standing posture too. Start this exercise slowly and move the head ten times each side in the beginning. Later, this can be increased to thirty times.

Side-ways movement

Now move the head sideways, stretching it as far as possible towards the right shoulder and then towards the left shoulder alternatively. Starting with 10 times, this movement can gradually be increased to 30 times.

Circular movement

Sit down if you are performing the above exercises in lying position. Move the neck in a circle, first from left towards right side (anticlockwise) and then from right towards left side in a circular motion. It should be done very slowly. The number of times this movement can be done is 10 times gradually increasing it to 30 times.

Special stretching of neck for strengthening thyroid gland

Apply some mustard oil or water on your right palm first. Now press it close to the left side of neck and stretch it to left side as far as it can go. Again do the same thing with your left palm and stretch towards right side. Repeat the exercises for at least ten times every day if not more.

Massage of neck for thyroid gland strengthening

Lubricate your palms with mustard oil and give a massage to your neck glands in a slow motion. First massage the neck muscles below the chin with hollow of your palms in upward direction, say for ten to fifteen times. Now massage the neck from left to right and then right to left. Next massage the muscles of the neck from back-side, left to right and then from right to left.

Sarvangasan (Stand on shoulders)

Although there is a name given to this, stand on shoulders asana but I am particularly mentioning the easy way so that people can understand the posture. It influences the whole body and its functions; the entire human organism. It has profound influence on *thyroid gland*. This asana gives exercise to the gland. Lie down on the floor and then raise both legs upwards with the help of both the hands in such a position that the hands are pressed on the back (above hips) and elbows/forearm rest on the floor. The body and the neck will make a ninety-degree angle in this pose. The chin will be touching the chest. Keep your eyes stuck to both thumbs of your feet. Hold this posture for some time according to capacity and bring back the legs to the ground very slowly without any jerks. The time of this posture can be increased according to the advice of master. As I told you earlier, there is always a need for a master to learn this art. This asana is one of the best for curing all thyroid diseases and has a special significance for the patients of *hyperthyroidism*.

Padmasan and Sidhasan

After getting up early in the morning preferably before the sunrise, finish your daily routine of toilet and cleaning teeth, etc. Now select a peaceful site where there is plenty of open air. Spread a clean mat over which you should take your seat. Fold your legs either in lotus asan (Padmasana) or Yoga mudra (Sidhasana). Sidhasana can be learnt from a person knowing yoga. For this, fold your left leg first onto your right thigh. Now fold the right leg over it. Or you can do the vice versa i.e. placing first right leg over the thighs and then the left leg over it. The heels will be beneath the navel region and the knees will be touching the earth. The soles of both the feet will be facing up. Keep your back in a straight posture and spread your hands on your knees. Now, fold the thumb and index finger of both the hands together, touching each other, leaving the rest three fingers of each hand spread on the knee. This asana is difficult but in due course of practice, it can be done with ease. If this is found a little difficult, you can try yoga mudra. For attaining Padmasana, place your left leg-heel beneath right thigh so that the heel touches the middle area between anus and genitals. Now put your right leg over it in such a manner that the sole of right foot faces up. Now place your hands on your lap, on the heel of the right leg. The hands are to be kept one above the other facing up. Please note that the heels of the legs should not be kept over the genitals. This is much easier asana and can be a starter for doing '*pranayama*'. Pranayama is the process of breathing smoothly, inhailing and exhaling from the nostrils as per the prescribed procedure.

Halasan

This asana is a continuation of Sarvangasan. First, observe the same posture as that of Sarvangasan and then bring your legs down towards your head side placing your feet on the floor behind your head. Thus you make an arch with the earth. The hands that were holding your back in 'sarvangasan' are to be placed straight on the earth. This asana has a special significance to cure patients of *hypothyroidism* and of course, it is good for all thyroid diseases. It activates the working of thyroid gland.

Vajrasan, sitting straight on folded legs

This asana is not exactly related with thyroid diseases but has a special effect on what you eat i.e. *metabolism*. It is very simple and one should do it regularly after the meals and in the morning. Fold your legs beneath the hips so that you sit on your soles, which in turn press the hips. Sit straight and place your palms on the knees. Sit like this for about five minutes after lunch and dinner and you will find your digestion improved, your memory sharpened and your menstruation regularized (females). Besides, it is very beneficial for knee pain.

Supta-vajrasan, lying on your folded legs and arms

Take your posture of vajrasan as stated above. Now, slowly lie down on the floor and this will make your both knees come together and soles coming outside the hips. Fold your arms beneath your head so that the left hand palm touches and comes beneath your right shoulder and your right hand palm comes beneath your left shoulder. The head will now be positioned on the cross of both your hands. This asana is performed with some difficulty and needs guidance of a master. Once it is learned and practiced, it is a guarantee against any diseases occurring due to malfunction of glands. *All the glands of the body are strengthened by this very asana. This asana is one of the best for thyroid gland diseases.*

These are few simple yoga exercises meant exclusively for curing thyroid diseases. There are many other asanas and postures to keep you fit and healthy and the same can be learned gradually.

STRESS AND THYROID CONNECTION

The ancient Indian culture and its natural methods of conducting Yoga is being revitalized in India in modern times. Now the actual awareness about yoga is capturing the attention of Europe and American states. In USA, a Mind Body Institute has been established and many Americans are doing research work there to find out the originality of our art and uses of this art to eliminate the diseases of both body and mind. Dr. Herbert Benson of this Institute has been doing research on stress. In his views, stress affects the central nervous system in such a way that it gives rise to diseases like hypertension, hypotension, irregular menstruation, arthritis, skin diseases, constipation, heart diseases and other tension related diseases. Naturally, thyroid disease might have been included being stress related. On 'stress, cause and results', a conference was held under the guidance of WHO in London wherein stress has been declared as one of the most carved out fatal disease.

There have been sufferers of stress disease right from the olden times and for this reason only, the art of *meditation* was developed. There has been a degree of variation in stress diseases in different ages. Even children are not free from stress these days due to higher involvement of mental work in schools and less of physical exercise due to the advent of television and computers. According to study, 12 out of 20 persons suffer from high stress every day in their routine business and jobs at home or at their working place and the rest 8 out of 20 suffer from normal stress. During the period of stress, our brain is severely affected and gets imbalanced. The hypothalamus section of our brain gets excited and then it activates the cortex part of the brain. Conflicting waves start flowing through the body. The pituitary gland starts secreting certain redundant hormones, which in turn convert biochemicals into toxic components. The ultimate result is depression, lethargy and restlessness.

Stress relieving Yogasanas

Shavasan (corpse pose)

Lie flat on your back on the floor and spread your feet keeping them at a distance of about two feet. Place a small pillow or folded blanket behind your head. Do not use a thick pillow. Your hands should be close to your body, touching the body. The palms should face upwards and hands should not be clenched. Close your eyes. Now feel relaxed and let your body be released or let loose. Try to feel the different parts of your body in contact with the floor.

For doing this, close your eyes and imagine that your entire body, part by part, is in touch with ground and is getting heavy. Do not get worried over this when you actually feel the limbs heavy. Throughout the practice of this asana, the worries and problems may keep cropping in or keep appearing. Convince and tell yourself that these problems will receive your attention after a few minutes and that you are now practicing shavasana. Gently and slowly you will gain confidence and you will feel relaxed in all respects. During the whole process of this asana, feel free and relaxed as if you are dead so far as your body is concerned. Remain in this position for some time, say at least ten minutes without any movement. While you are acting like a corpse, breathe deeply and take long breaths.

Ardhavajrasan

Sit on your knees, folding your legs backwards so that the feet are under your hips. Sit erect and now keep your both hands on the knees while your feet are together. This is *vajrasan*, which is beneficial for your digestion. We have already detailed this asana. Keeping this asana intact, now raise the both hands over your head and bend forward while breathing out. Bend slowly so that your head touches the ground and stretch your hand on the ground. Next step is to return to your initial position while breathing in. This is *ardhavajrasan*. One should repeat this bending and sitting-erect positions for five to ten times.

Pavanmuktasan

Sleep on the ground in 'shavasan' posture in a relaxed way. Bend both the knees with your hands and bring the knees close to your stomach. Hold your knees with your hands and breathe out forcefully. Now return to your initial position while breathing in. Repeat this for five to ten minutes. As the name indicates, this asana relieves gastric trouble and flatulence.

Shavsan is one of the best asanas for relief in stress. Dr. Datey, a renowned heart specialist of Mumbai and recipient of Dhanvantri award appreciates shavasan for releasing tensions. Explaining as to what happens when there is stress, he says, "There is at once an impulsive reaction. Stress is communicated to the brain by the five senses. *Thalamus* further transmits the impulse throughout the autonomus nervous system. Impulses are modified through *shavasan*. The shavasan is the best form of relaxation. You would not react to a crisis as an average person would. The shavasan was once given to 47 patients with hypertension of various etiologies. A significant response was obtained in about 52 percent of the patients. (From old age to youth through Yoga by Siddhantalankar)

MEDITATION AND THYROID CONNECTION

A balance of hormones is what is needed for thyroid gland. Meditation is one of the methods by which balance in hormones can be achieved. Meditation infuses harmony and natural order in human life. It brings a sort of awakening with a kind of creative intelligence and life becomes peaceful. Once this is achieved, no disease can harm the body.

Meditation is a process of mind through which one achieves peace and tranquility. Sit on a mat, spread on the floor, folding your legs one over the other either in sarvangasan or just sit casually. Relax your muscles and just watch the surroundings. Keep your ears open to all the sounds of the environment for some time. This way you will be observing the external world. After some time, try to forget about the environment and bring your thoughts to the inner mind by closing your eyes. Try to note the thoughts; that are crossing your mind. Concentrate on your process of thoughts let them be connected to anything, domestic or professional. Do not try to avoid those thoughts. As and when the time passes, these thoughts will slowly diminish. You will now feel a distraction and a radical transformation will be approaching you. There will be increased relaxation now since your mind is flowing with various thoughts but your silence is keeping them in their deserved place in one corner of the mind. A store house of energy will start flowing from within and you will have a feeling of 'no-thought' after some time. A blank will come after some time of silence. This is one form of meditation.

Another form of meditation is still easy to perform. In this, you have to sit quiet and observe the sound of your breathing. Breathing is the movement of your energy or 'prana' or the life force, which has only two aspects, inhalation (a cold breath) and exhalation (a warm breath). Together they form a natural rhythm. Slowly, you will realize that the breathing process is cosmic, a sound-free sound called 'Aum'. Aum has two aspects, male and female. The male is 'hum' and female is 'so'. During inhalation, the female energy 'so' gets in and during exhalation, the male energy 'hum' gets out. Now instead of listening to the sound of breathing, feel as if 'so' and 'hum' are created out of breathing procedure. Listen to 'so-hum' and 'hum-so' sound through the breath. Your breathing will become quiet and spontaneous and you will go beyond thoughts. There will be no limitations felt and your consicousness will empty itself. Consciousness will now expand. Creative intelligence will start to operate in your mind, body and consciousness. All your problems will get faded in this process of meditation.

Thyroid gland is connected with the brain and it is the brain that commands the gland. Once brain or mind is in tranquil state and in the sea of vast feeling of quiteness, thyroid is likely to get impact of this quiteness; there will be a balance maintained between the two and that is what is needed. *Meditation should also be done under the guidance of a master of Yoga to get its full benefits.*

SECTION - 3

Thyroid Function Tests

WHY THE TESTS?

The first thing that the patient questions, "Why are the tests required?" The doctor, particularly the homoeopaths have to make the patient satisfied on this. The patients know that in other systems of medicines, the tests are needed but why in homoeopathy? This is a vital question. The patient has to be told that homoeopathy is not the old system clinging to old values. The symptoms of the disease are still vital but when the modern facilities are available to confirm the nature of disease, it is essential that the disease is diagnosed fully to start the medicine. There is another way to detail the patient on this aspect. If a patient is having stones in gall bladder or kidneys, it has to be confirmed. No symptomatic diagnosis is complete although we have all the symptoms but the presence of stones is vital for the doctor to know. Similarly, the nature of tumor has to be ascertained whether it is benign or malignant. If primary remedies are not reacting to the tumor favorably, it becomes the duty of the homoeopath to get the biopsy done so that a definite line of treatment is suggested before it is too late. Homoeopathy is now quite advanced and it has to take assistance of the modern clinical diagnostic tools.

In most of the cases, the patient of hypothyroidism or hyperthyroidism come to the shelter of homoeopathy after they have consulted allopathic system of medicine. They are on the daily intake of allopathic medicines, which they would not like to part with due to strict instructions of the allopath. Even if the patient has not taken shelter of allopathy and it is the first time that he or she has come to homoeopathy, it is the duty of the homoeopath to make him/her understand in short as to what is this disease and why the thyroid function tests are needed? This will assure the patient that he or she is in right hands. Here is how the patient can be detailed in short about the disease.

TELL THE PATIENTS THAT THE TESTS ARE DONE

- To determine whether the thyroid gland is working or functioning properly. An underactive thyroid gland (hypothyroidism) and an overactive thyroid (hyperthyroidism) present different set of symptoms as have been explained earlier in the definitions.
- To help evaluate an enlarged thyroid gland (goiter).
- To check the newborn babies for any congenital hypothyroidism because such condition can interfere with normal growth and development and can cause other problems if not discovered soon. Such problems relate to mental retardation and cretinism.
- To have a monitoring over the treatment of thyroid diseases.

TELL THE PATIENT ABOUT HYPOTHYROIDISM AND HYPERTHYROIDISM

Hypothyroidism is a condition, which develops when the thyroid gland does not produce enough hormones. Thyroid hormones regulate the way the body uses energy. Lack of thyroid hormones affects many systems of the body and can cause a wide range of complaints including constipation, cold, tiredness, dry skin, thinning or falling of hair, poor memory and weight gain. The most general cause of the disease is Hashimoto's thyroiditis, which occurs when the natural defense system or immune system produces antibodies. These antibodies destroy the thyroid tissue.

THYROID FUNCTION TESTS

If the conditions are just opposite to the symptoms detailed above, it is called hyperthyroidism. We are talking about the diseases in short and hence shall not go into details for the patient to know.

NOW TELL THE PATIENT ABOUT GENERAL TREATMENT

For hyperthyroidism, three methods of treatment are needed in allopathy.

1. **Radioactive iodine:** It is a common method used nowadays in USA and India to treat the people with Grave's disease, especially those women who are not pregnant and over 21 years of age. *Radioactive iodine often destroys the entire thyroid gland, and eventually 80 percent or more of those treated develop hypothyroidism.*

2. **Antithyroid medication:** This is the most common treatment preferred in the initial stage in Asia and U.S.A. About thirty to forty percent of people undergoing this treatment go into remission for prolonged periods after the medication is stopped. People are required to take the medication for one or two years and even more at times.

3. **Thyroidectomy:** Surgical removal of a part of the thyroid gland is done only in some cases when an enlarged thyroid makes swallowing and breathing difficult.

One of the above treatments in allopathy, the pregnant women or breast-feeding women cannot be treated with radioactive iodine because it may harm the fetus.

THE TESTS

1. **TSH test:** TSH test or serum thyotrophin is the most sensitive test to screen for hypothyroidism. We have detailed about hypothyroidism. Further tests for changes in the specific thyroid hormones may be needed to determine if the thyroid

gland is causing hyperthyroidism or there is another cause like problems with pituitary gland.
2. **Antithyroid antibody test:** It may be required to help diagnose Grave's disease and autoimmune thyroiditis.
3. **Radioactive thyroid scan and radioactive iodine uptake test:** These are similar tests used to evaluate why thyroid gland is overactive.
4. **CT Scan and MRI:** In addition to above, there may be a need for CT scan and MRI for eyes area in case of Grave's ophthalmopathy.

In the case of hyperthyroidism also, *American Thyroid Association, USA* recommends that adults, particularly women should be scanned for thyroid dysfunciton beginning at the age of 35 and every five years thereafter. Early and frequent screening may be too costly for some people and it recommends that TSH test is adequate for the purpose. Frequent screening is recommended for those who have risk factors or symptoms of hyperthyroidism.

TELL THE PATIENT ABOUT THE PROCEDURE OF TESTS

Now the patient has to be told that hypothyroidism is suspected and to confirm it pathological tests are needed for the blood. The tests are TSH and T4 measurement. In case the above two tests are found abnormal, the patient may have Hashimoto's thyroiditis for which antithyroid antibody test will be required which is thyroid ultrasound test and thyroid scan with radioactive iodine update test. In some cases, a blood test called the thyrotrophin releasing hormone (TRH) stimulation test is done to diagnose other rare forms of hypothyroidism (Caused by diseases affecting hypothalamus and pituitary gland). If hypothalamus or pituitary is affected a *computerized axial tomography or CT scan* or a *Magnetic resonance imagining or MRI* of the hypothalamus or pituitary gland may also be needed to probe into these areas of the brain.

In U.S.A., most of the new-born babies are tested for hypothyroidism to check the possibility of mental retardation. This is not done in India. In U.S.A., a procedure holds good that people older than 35 should get themselves screened for hypothyroidism every five years and people older than 70 must get themselves checked regularly. American Thyroid Association, USA, has recommended this.

The other guidelines by this association include tests for thyroid for women who are in their first three months of pregnancy. Those women who are suffering from hypothyroidism are advised to go in for tests at regular intervals to determine if the dosage of thyroid hormone medication is adequate in them. In the case of postpartum hypothyroidism, if the women complain of weak memory, depression and loss of concentration, they are advised to undergo tests and take medicines. The reason given by the association is that the patients may not feel any symptoms belonging to thyroid and take the milder symptoms of depression etc. The full symptoms do not become apparent until the illness has become more advanced.

TELL ABOUT GENERAL INFORMATION AS TO WHO IS WHO IN THE LABORATORY

It is very important that a patient knows why he is at the hospital when he goes to a private or government hospital and whom he should contact for thyroid function test. On the reception desk of the hospital, different branches and sections of hospital are displayed. One must read and understand those branches of medicines. In the case of a check up of thyroid, one should consult an endocrinologist. *Endocrinologist is a doctor specialized in the treatment of hormone problems.* Similarly, he should know that a *Cardiologist* is a doctor specialized in treatment of problems *relating to heart and blood vessels.* He should also know that a *Radiologist* is a doctor who is specialized in treatment of diseases through radiation from radioactive substances, examining of X-rays and writing reports on its scanning is his job. The person who takes the blood samples from the patients is known as *Phlebotomist*. This is now-a-days done by laboratory assistants. This type of general information helps the patient to know about the jobs to be done and from whom to get done.

HOW THE TESTS ARE DONE?

The first job required by the patient will be to give blood sample for conducting the tests.

- The person in-charge of taking blood will wrap an elastic band around the upper arm of the patient to temporarily stop the circulation or flow of blood through the veins in the arm. This sort of wrapping makes it easier to put a needle into a vein properly. The band is fixed so that the veins below the band get larger and do not collapse easily.
- The needle site is cleaned with spirit (alcohol) and the needle is inserted. Sometimes, there may be needed more than one insertion of needles because of the fact that needle does not get placed correctly or when veins cannot supply enough blood.
- After the needle is properly placed in the vein, a collection tube is attached to the needle. Now the blood will flow into the collection tube. At times, when it is felt that the quantity of blood is insufficient for tests, another tube may be attached to collect more blood.
- When enough blood is collected, the band around the arm is removed. A cotton ball or gauze pad is placed over the site of puncture as the needle is withdrawn from the vein. Pressure is applied to the site of puncture for some minutes and then a small bandage is often placed over it.
- The patient need not worry about the needle puncture

over the arm as it is just a prick. He or she may feel a sort of pinch or sting as the needle goes down the skin. When the needle is in the skin, some patients report a feeling of stinging but most of the patients do not feel so because the discomfort is negligible and almost painless. The amount of discomfort or pain depends upon the efficiency of the person who is taking the blood sample.

RISK FACTORS IN GIVING BLOOD FOR TESTS

- There is very little risk of complications from the above procedure. Some people develop a small bruise at the site of puncture. Keeping finger pressure on the site of puncture for several minutes, especially after the needle is withdrawn can reduce this risk of bruising.
- After the blood sample is taken from the arm of the patient, it is very rare that an inflammation occurs over the vein (phlebitis). In case this occurs, the easy way is to treat it with warm compress application several times daily.
- Patients, who have bleeding disorders, continuous bleeding could be a problem. Those who are in the habit of taking aspirin or other blood thinning tablets are prone to bleeding from the site of puncture. In case of any bleeding or clotting problems, it should be told to the doctor in advance before the blood sample is taken so that proper care is taken and medication is started in advance.

I have given details as to how the patient should be briefed so that they do not hesitate to get the tests done. The following are the pointers for the homoeopaths to know.

Coming to the thyroid function test, we measure the hormone levels of T3, T4 and TSH but before modern method of thyroid function test came into existence, the doctors were performing *'Radioactive Iodine'* test. In this test, an irradiated form of iodine was orally given and the level of radioactivity was measured using a special counter to examine the amount absorbed by the thyroid gland. Iodine is an essential part of thyroxine, a more rapid uptake than the normal could show over activity because the gland struggles to manufacture thyroxine. On the other hand, a less rapid than normal uptake suggests under activity. Now a days such tests are not performed.

ULTRASOUND—WHAT IS IT AND HOW IT IS DONE?

In order to check the size, texture and shape of the thyroid gland, different types of scanning is advised by some doctors. Ultrasound test is one of the common tests of which people are aware. In this test, high frequency sound waves are bounced off the gland to build up a picture on a small screen. To facilitate a better picture, a gel is rubbed on to the neck so that sound waves pass through it easily. A transducer (an instrument which converts sound waves into electrical signals) is passed over the neck.

RADIOISOTOPE SCANS

It is special type of X-ray to see the lump in the thyroid and check whether it is malignant or not. This test is also useful to see the structure of the thyroid and how it is working.

MRI AND CT TESTS

These are brain scan test and the people suffering from eye problems may need these tests. These test are performed if the doctor suspects that the problem has originated from the pituitary gland. *MRI is magnetic resonance imaging whereas CT is computed tomography.*

AUTOANTIBODY TEST

This is a blood test to check the presence of antibodies against the thyroid and it is conducted when there is doubt about autoimmune problems like Hashimoto and Grave's diseases. There are other antibodies like thyroid stimulating antibodies, which boost thyroid activity. Nine out of ten patients suffering from Grave's disease have it, while those in the early stage of Hashimoto's can have this problem of antibodies.

CELL EXAMINATION

We have talked about malignancy of the gland while discussing about radioisotope scan. Another method of diagnosis for cancer is examination of the cells. It is conducted through a fine needle aspiration, which enables the doctor to remove few cells from the thyroid gland and examine these under a microscope. It is a painless procedure and doctor uses a fine syringe to do this test in a few seconds. Now-a-days this has replaced the conventional biopsy in which a small piece of tissue is cut out for examination.

HORMONE LEVEL CONTRASTS

- If thyroid is over active (hyperthyroidism), T3 level is higher, T4 may also be higher but TSH level will be lowered in comparison with the normal values.
- If the thyroid is under active (hypothyroidism), T4 level is low, T3 may also be low but TSH will be high in comparison with the normal values.

OTHER LABORATORY TESTS

- *Basal Metabolic Rate:* Its normal value is 20 percent. It is elevated, say, plus 30-100 percent. Of course, this has become obsolete because of its various limitations. The test is estimated by finding out the oxygen consumption of the patient in the basal state. The reading thus obtained is compared with a normal standard and the difference is recorded as a percentage. The rate may vary from minus twenty to plus twenty percent. In toxic goiter, the rate is increased to plus eighty per cent and in myxedema, it is decreased to about minus forty five percent.

- *Protein Bound Iodine:* Its normal value is 3.5 to 8 µg per 100ml; an excess over 8 µg is found in most of the patients. It is increased to 10-15 µg percent. If the patient is pregnant, or has hepatitis, thyroiditis, iodine medication, mercurial diuretics and antithyroid drugs, the serum bound iodine may show a false rise.
- *Butanol Extractable Iodine:* It is raised to 8-14 µg percent whereas the normal values are 3-6.5. This is test not widely available.
- Plasma cholesterol is low, 100-140 mg percent. The normal is 150-250 percent.
- Electrocardiography shows a rapid rate with tall R and T waves, auricular fibrillation or flutter (occasional), left ventricular hypertrophy in late cases.
- Blood examination show relative lymphocytosis.
- Serum calcium is occasionally elevated.
- Urine examination will reveal slight glycosuria.
- In case of suppression test, when 65 mg of thyroid is administered thrice daily or triiodothyronine (70-150 µg) is administered daily for seven days, there should be no drop in 24 hours uptake of radioactive iodine. In normal persons, there will be 30 percent drop.
- Few cases of hyperthyroidism (T3 toxicosis) are on account of excessive production of T3 without any associated rise in the level of serum PBI or the serum T4.
- The T4 that is free in the serum and not protein bound show the level of hormones available to the individual thyroid cell than is the total serum T4.
- *Blood cholesterol level* falls in hyperthyroidism and rises in hypothyroidism.
- *Serum creatinine* in blood is higher than 0.6 mg per 100 ml in case of thyrotoxicosis even if the BMR is not raised.

[**Note:** *Clinical features of thyrotoxicosis, Grave's disease and exophthalmic goiter have many similarities and it is the different clinical tests, which would identify and limelight the name of the particular disease.*]

MEASURING THYROID HORMONES IN THE SERUM

The following serum type are tested:
1. Serum protein bound iodine (PBI).
2. Total serum thyroxine i.e. T4.
3. Total serum tri-iodo-thyronine i.e. T3.
4. Free serum thyroxine i.e. T4.
5. Free serum tri-iodo-thyronine i.e. T3.

T3 and T4 hormones having iodine are carried in the plasma mainly by a specific binding protein, thyroxine binding globulin (TBG), and by thyroxine binding prealbumin. Because very small amounts of T3 and T4 are free in the blood, PBI effectively indicates total circulating thyroid hormones. As per the book, 'Bailey & Love's Short Practice Of Surgery' (1975), the state of normal thyroid function (euthyroid) has a range of 3.5 to 8 µg/100ml and normal range for T4 total serum is 3.0 to 7.5 µg/100ml. Total serum T3 and free serum T4 are measured by radio-immuno assay.

MEASURING FREE OR UNOCCUPIED BINDING SITES FOR THYROID HORMONES IN THE BLOOD

In the T3 uptake test, radioactive T3 is incubated with the patient's serum so that it becomes fixed to any thyroid binding protein not already carrying T3 or T4. The amount so fixed can be measured and from this can be estimated the number of binding sites in the serum which are unoccupied.

In hyperthyroidism, the number of free binding sites is low and in hypothyroidism, the number of the free sites is high. Taking use of Thyopac method, the mean normal value is assumed as 100 percent for free binding sites. A figure of 85 percent or less suggests hyperthyroidism whereas a figure of 120 percent or more suggests hypothyroidism. Thyopac is not a very accurate test but in conjunction with the total serum T4 or the serum PBI, the Free Thyroxine Index (F.T.I.) can be calculated by a fixed formula.

VIVO TEST (DISCHARGE AND UPTAKE OF IODINE BY THYROID GLAND) AND OTHER MISCELLANEOUS TESTS

1. The radioactive iodine uptake test

The way our thyroid treats the inorganic iodine in our body makes no differentiation while treating the radioactive isotopes of iodine. Accordingly, when a smallest dose (trace dose) is given to the patient, it is rapidly absorbed from the small bowel into the blood and the kidneys and the thyroid rush for it, rather compete for it. In hyperthyroidism, the thyroid uptake is rapid and a little is excreted in the urine. The isotopes get embedded into the T3 and T4 molecules and pass back into the serum. They can be measured as Protein Bound Iodine (PBI). *A quick uptake of iodine and a quick turnover indicate hyperthyroidism. (There is a fixed rate of hours for this calculation)*

Iodine uptake test has been very nicely explained in the book, 'Clinical Methods in Surgery' by K. Das. It is easy to understand:

"The funciton of the thyroid gland is better understood by its capacity to concentrate iodine (10,000 times more than other tissues). The patient who has not received any iodine medication for at least one month, is given a tracer quantity of radioactive iodine (i.e. 25 microcuries in 100 ml of water for a normal-sized gland, the dose should be increased when the gland is larger than normal) and the uptake is directly measured by Geiger-Muller counter 24 hours after the dose imbibed. In healthy subjects, the iodine uptake is about 20-40% i.e. this amount is retained by the thyroid gland and the rest is excreted. *An uptake of 55% or more indicates hyperthyroidism and the uptake of 20% or less indicates hypothyroidism.*"

Precautions for the patients undergoing radioactive iodine test

Radioactive iodine test is supposed to be safe for sufferers of thyroid overactivity but this test can affect the thyroid function of people with normal thyroid. This problem of after effect of the test for patients having normal thyroid can be cleared by isolating the patient for a week or so in the hospital until the dose has cleared from the system (body).

Patients who are treated with lower doses or tested for the second time or subsequent time, can go to their homes but in that case also, a care has to be taken to make minimum contacts with people. Not much of time should be spent in public places and a distance should be kept from the children and members of the family. Keep distance from babies and avoid kissing them. There should not be any close contact with husband or wife until the radioactivity has cleared from the system.

Taking this test is sometimes traumatic for some patients. They develop diarrhea and sickness with nose bleeding or sore gums. Depression and anger are most common features after the test. To avoid this sort of condition of mind, one should engage in reading some good books or spend time in viewing video films.

2. T3 suppression test (Werner)

In the case of a toxic goiter, which is eager to absorb iodine because of its iodine deficiency in endemic areas, there is a rapid iodine uptake when given. A simple goiter is under TSH control so suppressing the TSH production can diminish that uptake. This is accomplished by giving 40 µg of T3 (triiodothronine) to the patient for seven days at the interval of eight hours and the results watched on a graph curve. Radio-iodine uptake curves are compared before and after T3 suppression when a toxic goiter may show up to 10 to 20 percent reduction in uptake while a simple goiter will show 50 to 80 percent reduction. In difficult cases of diagnosing thyrotoxicosis, this test is useful. Also it is useful in assessment of ophthalmic Grave's disease where the patient may have normal thyroid function (euthyroid) but uptake of radio-iodine is not suppressed.

3. Scanning of thyroid

After the patient is given a tracer dose of iodine, if the thyroid is scanned, one can see which parts of the gland are functioning or not functioning (hot or cold). Such a scanning is most useful in diagnosis of an autonomous toxic nodule, be it a solitary toxic nodule or as a part of a toxic multinodular goiter. The malignancy part of the goiter can also be visualized.

4. Protein Bound Plasma Activity

The patient, who has not been given iodine for atleast two weeks, is fed a dose of 10-20 microcuries of radioactive iodine and 10 ml of blood is taken 48 hours later. In case of renal diseases, the test conducted may indicate a false high reading. So this test should be excluded for renal disease sufferers. The normal range is 0 to 0.4% of dose found in one liter of plasma. In thyrotoxicosis, it is more than 0.4%.

5. Laryngoscopy

It is helpful in diagnosing involvement of the recurrent laryngeal nerve.

6. Radiography

It is of great help in diagnosing the position of the trachea, which may be displaced or depressed by the goiter. X-ray taking is also helpful in diagnosing a retrosternal goiter. If the thyroid gland is malignant in nature X-ray of the bones (especially of the skull) suspected to be secondarily involved should be done for evidence of metastasis.

THYROID FUNCTION TESTS

FACTORS THAT AFFECT THE RESULTS OF THE TESTS

- The medication can interfere with thyroid function test result. This medication may be use of corticosteroids and hormones such as estrogen, progestrone and birth control pills. Drugs intake like levodopa (larodopa), dopamine, lithium (eskalith, lithonate), methimazol (tapazole) and propylthiouracil can affect the results of tests.
- Heavy or large doses of aspirin before the test.
- Medicines like Ideral, betachron, tegretol, coumadin, dilantin, eskalith, lithonate and atromid etc.
- Pregnancy can also affect thyroid function tests results. In this case, TSH level may be low.
- Contrast material used for certain X-ray imaging tests may affect T4 results.
- Long term chronic illness and stress therein can interfere with the results of tests.
- Rough handling, inadequate refrigeration or contamination of blood sample while storing or handling can cause inaccurate test results.

GENERAL OBSERVATION

TSH test is supposed to be most useful for the conditions that can affect the thyroid gland.

Generally physicians consider the result of thyroid hormone tests, especially T4 results when checking with the results of TSH.

There is another test, which measures TSH level in the blood. This is called thyrotrophin releasing hormone challenge test or TRH. In this test, TSH blood levels are measured before and after an injection of TRH. The injection causes the pituitary gland to release TSH. With the injection, if the TSH levels do not rise, it indicates conditions like damage to the pituitary gland or Grave's disease.

Importance of Thyroid Function Tests

THE PATIENT coming from the system of allopathic medicine generally bring his report on function tests and treat it as a religious document to confirm the extent of disease. It is this document, which is advised from time to time to check the gravity of the disease, be it hypothyroidism or hyperthyroidism. Basically physicians see three major measurements i.e. T4, T3 and TSH.

THYROXINE—T4

Most of the T4 in blood is attached to a protein called thyroxine-binding globulin. Less than one percent of the T4 is unattached. This is called free T4 or FT4 and it affects the metabolism. The amount of FT4 can be measured. However, it is more common to measure the total T4 amount.

TRIIODOTHYRONINE—T3

T3 has more of effect than T4 in the body. T3 is present in the metabolism in lower amount than T4 and yet it works efficiently. The reason is that of T3 is made from T4 by the body tissues after T4 is released from the thyroid gland. The rest of T3 is produced by the thyroid gland itself. The total amount of T3 in the blood or the amount of free T3 (FT3) can be measured. As a general rule, less than one percent of the T3 is free.

THYROID STIMULATING HORMONE—TSH

We have already discussed and learnt about the definition of T4 and T3 under the hormone study (page 19). Regarding TSH, it is a hormone, which triggers the thyroid to make its own hormones, thyroxin (T4) and triiodothyronine (T3). These help to control the body's use of food for energy or metabolism. A TSH test measures the amount of TSH in the blood and is considered the most reliable method of detecting a thyroid problem.

We know that hormones are required for normal development of the brain. This is very essential in the first three years of life. If a child lacks in the efficient working of thyroid gland and his or her gland is not producing enough thyroid hormone i.e. congenital hypothyroidism, there are chances that the child may have mental retardation.

The production of TSH is through release of a substance by hypothalamus. This substance is called thyrotopin-releasing hormone. It is this hormone, which triggers the pituitary gland to release TSH or thyroid stimulating hormone.

To find out the efficiency of the gland with respect to TSH in particular, some tests are conducted. An underactive thyroid gland can cause symptoms such as weight gain, tiredness, dry skin and constipation etc. Such a condition with above symptoms is called **hypothyroidism**. On the other hand, symptoms like weight loss, rapid heart rate, nervousness, diarrhea and feeling of being too hot etc. amount to the disease called **hyperthyroidism**.

The low or high levels of above hormones are decided after comparing with the normal range. There are many fluctuations in their levels due to different influences like pregnancy, drugs and emotional factor. However, measuring the value of level of TSH is sensitive test for primary thyroidism because it starts to rise before T4 falls below the lower limit and it is vice versa. TSH and thyroid hormones have two different and opposite conditions. When one is raised, the other is lowered and vice versa.

It may, therefore, be noted that hyperthyroid and hypothyroid both have a common bearing to check and that is TSH. It is the value, which shows as to how well the thyroid is working.

INCREASED LEVELS OF TSH

A high thyroid stimulating hormones (TSH) test result shows an underactive thyroid gland caused by failure of the thyroid gland. This can be called primary thyroidism and it is due to thyroiditis.

A higher TSH value can also occur in persons with an underactive thyroid gland especially such persons who are receiving too little thyroid hormone medication.

In rare cases, a high TSH value can occur from a pituitary gland tumor that is producing excess amounts of TSH. In such a case, a patient may have symptoms of hyperthyroidism.

DECREASED LEVELS OF TSH

As stated earlier, a low thyroid stimulating hormone or TSH value amounts to overactive thyroid (hyperthyroidism). The reason for hyperthyroidism is Grave's disease, a kind of goiter which may be multinodular or a benign (non-cancerous) tumor called a toxic nodule.

When there is low value of TSH, there can be damage to the pituitary gland, which prevents it from producing TSH. When this happens, it is called secondary hypothyroidism. In such a case, the symptoms are tiredness, weight gain, dry skin and constipation with a feeling of being too cold or frequent menstrual periods.

A low value of TSH can also occur in patients with an underactive thyroid gland and these are those patients who are receiving too much thyroid hormone medication.

VALUES OF THYROID FUNCTION TEST

Normal values or range for levels of T3, T4 and TSH mostly depends upon the average level found in a slice of the normal population and there is a variation from region to region. Reference ranges of the hormone level in India, USA and UK are as follows:

U.K.	U.S.A
T4: 50-160 nmol/1.	T4: 5-12, Free thyroxine FT4: 0.9-2.4
T3: 1.0-2.9 nmol/1.	T3: 70-195 ng/dl. Free triiodothronine : 0.2-0.6 ng/dl.
TSH: 0.5-5.5 mU/L	Free thyroxine index, FTI: 4-11, TSH: 0.4-5 ml U/L (adults) and 3-20 ml U/L (new born)

NORMAL VALUES OF THYROID FUNCTION TESTS IN INDIA (VARIOUS LABORATORIES*)

*The above figures on the normal values of thyroid function tests are for the purpose of illustration because the exact figures may vary slightly from laboratory to laboratory.

(Important Note: Normal values may vary from lab to lab)

Institute of Nuclear Medicines and Allied Sciences, Delhi	T3: 70 to 220 ng/dl T4: 4.5 to 13.5 ug/dl TSH: 0.25 to 5.0 u.i. U/ml
A laboratory in Pathankot, hilly areas (JK)	T#: 0.75 to 2.1 ng/ml T4: 4.7 to 11 µg/dl T3: 0.5 to 2.5 U/ml
A laboratory in Srinagar hilly areas (JK)	T4: 0.5 to 13 µg/dl TSH: 0.4 to 7.0 u.i. U/ml
A popular laboratory of C. Place, New Delhi	**T3 free: 2.3 to 4.20 pg/ml **T4: free −0.89 to 1.80 ng/ml TSH: 0.49 to 4.67 u.i.U/ml

A laboratory in Ghaziabad (UP)	**T3 free: 1.4 to 4.4 ng/dl **T4 free: 0.8 to 2.0 ng/ml TSH: 0.2 to 2.0 m.i.U. /ml
A famous laboratory of Khanpur, New Delhi	T3: 1.64 to 3.45 pg/ml T4: 0.71 to 1.85 ng/ml TSH: 0.5 to 5.0 u.i.U/ml
A reliable laboratory in Faridabad (Haryana) ***TSH: 0.5 to 5.0 u.i.U/ml	T3: 1.64 to 3.45 pg/ml T4: 0.71 to 1.85 ng/ml
Escorts Hospital and Research Center, Faridabad (Haryana)	Elisa thyroid profile T3: 0.5 to 2.5 ng/ml T4: 0.5 to 13 µg/dl TSH: 0.4 to 7.0 u.i.U/ml
A reliable laboratory in Jaipur (Rajasthan)	T3: 0.7 to 2 ng/ml T4: 5.5 to 13.5 µg/dl TSH: 0.2 to 6.5 u.i.U/ml
A reputed laboratory Patna (Bihar)	Elisa thyroid profile T3: 0.75 to 2.1 ng/ml T4: 4.7 to 11.1 µg/dl TSH: 0.3 to 4.0 u.i.U/ml
A famous laboratory in Mumbai (Maharashtra)	T3: 70 to 200 ng/100 ml T4: 5 to 13 µg/100 ml TSH: 1to . u.i.U/ml

**Now-a-days it is very common to test the fraction of thyroxine not bound to the proteins that carry it around the bloodstream, which is thus called 'free thyroxine'. It is either a first line test or if the total thyroxine level is abnormal. Free thyroxine is mostly raised in hyperthyroidism and reduced in hypothyroidism. There is still an argument as to which is the best method of measuring free T4 and the validity of results with some methods of testing. There is one more important factor which influences the test reports as to their normal values. Thyroid hormone levels are subject to many different influences including pregnancy stage, use of pills to avert pregnancy and use of the drugs for some other diseases.

***TSH measurement is obviously a sensitive test for primary hypothyroidism. TSH starts to rise before T4 falls below the lower limit. Similarly, very high sensitive TSH tests show suppression of TSH before thyroid hormone levels are sufficiently raised in hyperthyroidism.

Note: µg, ng, ml, dl and u.i.U are units of measuring the values. mU/L is the measuring unit adopted in USA and it means milli-international units per liter. In order to conform to SI units, cell counts are to expressed/lit. The general formula for calculation of conversion factor from ng/dl to mol/L is ng/dl X 10 X 1000 mol/m^3 depicts volume and mol/S states chemical reaction. Sometimes, introducing of SI units is impractical as in the case of volume; liter as a unit is more convenient. SI units have not been widely adopted and hence older units have been retained.

Role of Homoeopathy

WE HAVE heard people saying that he or she has thyroid problem and most of the times, these people complain of chorea, decrease in weight, restlessness and palpitation. No one could think of thyroid problem and consider the above symptoms as debility, anaemia or some cardiac problem but when the tests are done and the doctor notes the other symptoms, the thyroid problem is detected. Just opposite to these conditions, a patient complains of increase in weight, dryness of skin and restlessness, he is also told that he or she has thyroid problem after the tests confirm it. Take another case where thyroid is again affected. There is a tumor like protrusion coming on the neck just below the face. Doctor is consulted and the patient is told that he has thyroid problem. So, in general terms all these conditions although opposing each other, are nothing but thyroid problems. All these variations are due to excessive or decreased flow of hormone thyroxine and these variations produce different symptoms.

We, the homoeopaths, have a significant example of this disease to quote if someone says that name of disease matters and symptoms do not. We need not know the name of the disease, say hypothyroidism, hyperthyroidism, thyroiditis, goiter and so on. We have discussed this in detail in the first section of the book. It was necessary to know the history of the diseases connected with thyroid before homoeopathy is brought into light.

We have already discussed about the climatic and regional land conditions under which the disease gets the lever to raise its head in the population. This factor is not to be forgotten when we treat a patient from say, Jammu and Kashmir, Himachal, Laddakh or north east states of the Himalayan territory.

A simple swelling existing for a longer time on the thyroid gland can be called goiter but again we have to go by symptoms of the body. The first visible symptom is swelling and other symptoms will themselves declare the name of the disease and like-wise remedy. In the other related diseases of thyroid, there need not be any swelling like that of goiter.

It is the name of this wonderful therapy, Homoeopathy, which attracts most of the person suffering from thyroid problems not because they know the meaning and fruitfulness of homoeopathy but because they want to get rid of the medicines of the orthodox system that had been prescribed when the patients were say, 28 years old. At the age of forty, they thought of switching over to Homoeopathy because they felt that continuous intake of Eltroxin might produce some worse effects. It is the firm thinking in India that the old medicinal system of Unani, Ayurveda, or Hakims are the real healers.

In such an atmosphere, people in rural India still go for allopathy more than the other systems of medicines because of the facilities provided by the government in each remote region. The pain killers, the ointments, the cough syrups are so much advertised on DD channels of TV (cable is distant dream for common public in villages) that even a child can fetch medicine for headache from the village chemist and give it to his grandfather who is busy playing cards under the shade of a tree and never wanted a tablet merely on a reason that he spoke of slight headache to his grandson. Any severe pain of any origin is supposed to be eliminated by a prick of needle (Injection), so says a villager. Allopathy has such a wide publicity network that Ayurveda, the system with traditional-belief of benefits, cannot dream of competing allopathy, leave aside homoeopathy. Homoeopathy has not reached the masses because the actual masses (about eighty percent of whole population of India) are in the rural areas and homoeopathy is still in the budding stage to extend its arms towards villages. During my stay in Bengal, Bihar and Assam, I have seen people drawn towards homoeopathy and if any revolution is likely to come for adopting homoeopathy in rural India, it will start from the eastern side. If you are practicing in Punjab or Haryana, you must have observed that many persons hailing from Bengal and Bihar come to you to enquire about the availability of homoeopathic medicines. Bengalis in particular, have very fair knowledge of medicines of homoeopathy and they do not hesitate to keep in stock at home a bottle of Arnica or Belladonna for their children in case of an injury or fever.

Thyroid disease is not commonly diagnosed, be it hypo or hyperthyroidism, in rural India. Upon a swelling in the neck, the word, "Ghengha" (goiter) is used for the disease. No villager goes for homoeopathy even in the case of goiter. There are many elderly people in the village, who take charge of the upkeep of health in respect of their village-brothers. It is they who suggest them to go to cities for the treatment of goiter, if the local medication of a 'Vaidya' and 'Hakim' in the village is unable to control the growth of goiter.

During my posting in the rural areas and jungles of Bihar, Orissa, Assam, Manipur and Bhutan, I have seen many patients with goiter. Here in these states, I have observed that Homoeopathy has an upper edge over Ayurveda, if not Allopathy. In West Bengal town of Siliguri, the hill areas of Bengal, Sikkim and Bhutan bring in many patients of this disease to the plains like Siliguri where there are many popular homoeopaths. I have observed this during my stay (1987-89) and also dealt with some cases of goiter in Bhutan (Nanglam village). Goiter, to me, was one of the prime causes to bring Homoeopathy in limelight in the area. "If homoeopathy can cure goiter, there is no reason why other acute diseases cannot be looked after" was the belief of the people.

In the towns and cities of North India, the cases of goiter are less due to serious awareness about the disease and emphasis by the government through wide publicity. It is strange enough that cases of thyroid diseases are found more among females in the urban areas. Leave aside goiter, the other diseases of the thyroid do exist there but are not brought to front due to non-availability to test facilities and lack of awareness among both people and the doctors. Symptoms of thyroid disease go on leading to names of different diseases until the persistency compels a competent doctor to advise for thyroid function tests. First of all, even if the doctor prescribes the thyroid tests, the people avoid it because it is costly and a rare test for a common man. The test is rare in the sense that it is not done in clinics of small towns and villages. Stool, urine or blood tests or even X-ray, ECG and sonography are the test well known to the public but thyroid tests are not familiar to the public.

So, in view of the above analogy, no one can say that thyroid diseases do not exist in villages. These do exist but are not diagnosed.

Coming back to our subject, it is well established that once thyroid test is done, there is every possibility that the patient will be prescribed medication for a lifetime. This compels the patient to opt for homoeopathy, not that homoeopathy will cure them but due to a hope of recovery. It is normal tendency of a person to have biased feeling about allopathic medication due to its side effects. No amount of consolation will deter a patient to search for alternative therapy so that he or she can get rid of allopathic medicine. The role of homoeopathy starts in the same manner as in resorting to homoeopathy for treatment of multiple warts, corns and renal or gall bladder stones, provided there is awareness about the competency of homoeopathy. I have seen many allopaths advising their patients to go in for a trial in homoeopathy in the case of warts and kidney stones. It is a fact that it takes much more time to cure a thyroid disease than eliminating a wart or expulsion of calculi from kidneys. Patients of thyroid diseases, once convinced about the results, shall never leave you till you tell them to stop the medicine. Sometimes, homoeopathic treatment becomes a sort of alternative compulsion on the part of the patient especially if the patient had experienced cure in skin or kidney diseases himself. Come what may, the patient desires to get rid of the daily dose of allopathic medicine and for this homoeopathy is one of the best and cannot be ignored.

THE HELP OF HOMOEOPATHY

The first duty of a homoeopath is to assure the patient that homoeopathic treatment will certainly make a dent in the followed procedure of the patients and betterment is surely expected. The main worry of the patient is that he has to take the allopathic medicines throughout his life and to avoid this only the patient has come to the shelter of homoeopathy. It is the duty of a homoeopath to make the patient understand that this is possible in this discipline. For achieving the confidence of the patient, the doctor has to make a brief speech on the system of homoeopathy as to how it works. The patient has to be told in the following fashion:

THEORY OF HOMOEOPATHY FOR A LAYMAN

"Health is a state of balance and the disease is the result of weakness of the body's energy or vital force or the 'Aatmik Shakti'. Once the vital force gets diminished, the body reflects the same in any of the diseases and one of them is thyroid disorder. The treatment is, therefore, aimed at strengthening the vital force so that the body itself heals the ailment. The symptoms of the disease are main features over which the medicines are selected. The remedies are based upon the law that substances which produce some symptoms when given to a healthy person, will cure the same symptoms if given to a diseased person. The principle is 'like cures like' (law of similars). The remedies are made from herbs, plants, minerals, animals and other substances. The substances are repeatedly diluted, shaken or succused by which the power of the substance is increased or call it that the substances are potentized. Potentization is nothing but increasing the invisible power of the substances. This sort of invisible power or energy stimulates the weak vital force because of the fact that it is of the same nature of which the patient suffers. It will nourish the vital force and restore the body to harmony. A homoeopath selects the remedy after checking with symptoms of the body and name of the disease is of no use to him. It is these symptoms, which enables him to choose the right remedy. If a thyroid patient has ill temper, irritable behavior, talks very fast, has red, wild and staring eyes and can not stand the sun-heat and his face has a red color, his remedy is *Belladonna*.

Belladonna is a good remedy for an overactive thyroid. But this is not all, every person has a different remedy because different people have different symptoms. If the patient has above symptoms but lacks in thirst and is very restless or has his tongue with a white coating, the remedy will differ. Similarly, if a patient having urticaria has no thirst and a patient having the same disease has thirst with restlessness, the remedy will differ although the name of the disease is same i.e. urticaria (*Apis* and *Rhus-t.*). In thyroid problems or in any disease, the whole base is symptoms and it is upon the skill of the homoeopaths to understand and interpret the symptoms and select a remedy."

You will find that there is a great impact of this sharing of ideas between the homoeopath and the patient. Give enough time to the patient so that he or she feels that your intention to cure is most important and hence all this explanation about the theory of the discipline.

THE PATIENT HAS TO BE TOLD THE ADVANTAGE OF HOMOEOPATHY

- Homoeopathy is safe and with minimum side effects, if occurring. First of all there would not be any side effects.
- It harnesses the self-regulating mechanism of cure of the whole body and not only the part of body being treated.
- It addresses the root-cause of the problem of body.
- It is quite effective and safe.
- It can be used along with the other medication of allopathy (Eltroxine etc. till weaned out).
- It fits into the life style of the patient and there are not many restrictions like taking of onions, garlic, coffee or wearing scents etc.
- It is comparatively less expensive.

Besides above, the patient has to be told that there is a limitation in allopathic system of medicines. Allopathy is geared towards treatment of symptoms only. It does not go deep into the root or the intrinsic cause of the disease. The treatment is, therefore, limited to one aspect and as soon as the symptoms vanish, the treatment ends. After sometime, a relapse may occur and symptoms further appear. On the other hand, Homoeopathy goes deep into the root of the disease considering into account all the factors, which led to the disease. These factors are various ranging from the cause of disease, psychological condition, tensions, anxiety, modalities and fatigue and so on.

There is a very fine example, which can be quoted to the patient. In case of a headache, one can take aspirin and headache goes away. What was the cause of this headache is not known to the conventional system of medicine till tests are done and who goes for tests for simple headaches. If the same case goes to the homoeopath, he will enquire for about an hour to find out the life history, hereditary aspects, food-habits, and modalities and so on before finding out a remedy. This means he wants to go deep into the cause of headache. Is it due to weak eyesight, sinusitis, wrong diet, constipation or anxiety? This all has to be taken into account and hence homoeopathic remedies once selected give foolproof cure.

CASE TAKING IN THYROID DISEASES

There is nothing special while taking a case of thyroid diseases. In each case, there has to be complete agreement with the procedure laid down by the great master in aphorism 84 of the Organon. This has been fully explained by J.T. Kent in his book 'Lectures on Homoeopathic Philosophy'. Here is my interpretation:

HOW TO RECORD A CASE?

Case taking of the thyroid-disease patient needs a lot of experience and training. This cannot be achieved by reading books only because the books will only provide basic knowledge and the method to take up the case. This means the process of knowledge will be in terms of rules. The actual learning comes by training from an experienced homoeopath after a complete degree in homoeopathy. Initially one has to watch the proceedings of taking up acute and chronic cases, note down the impressions and then comes the questions and clarification to be asked for from the trainer homoeopath. One has to interpret the uttering of the patient and conclude the symptoms as narrated by the patient. This, once written in one's own language needs a checking by the trainer. The main goal of the interview of the patient is to reach totality of symptoms. To reach this goal needs lot of time, effort and skill. Homoeopathic case taking is indeed an art.

Hahnemann has detailed the case taking in aphorism 100 in a very sensible manner as follows:

"...The novelty or peculiarity of a disease of that kind makes no difference either in the mode of examining or of treating it, as the physician must any way regard the pure picture of every prevailing disease as if it were something new and unknown, and investigate it thoroughly for itself, if he desired to practice medicine in a real and radical manner, never substituting conjecture for actual observation, never taking for granted that the case of disease before him is already wholly or partially known, but always carefully examining it in all the phases." (Organon of Medicine, S. Hahnemann)

Now read this statement and you will be aware that the prescriber should never be prejudiced. Dr. J.T. Kent, in his book, 'Lectures on Homoeopathic Philosophy' elaborates on aphorism 100 of his master Hahnemann. What a great contribution Kent has made towards the rules of Homoeopathy in his own language interpreting the aphorisms in his novel method so that the followers get a clear picture of what Hahnemann intends to say. Here is Kent's summary of aphorisms 100.

"Keep that in your mind, underscore it half a dozen times with red ink, paint it on the wall, put an index finger to it. One of the most important things is to keep out of the mind, in an examination of the case, some other case that has appeared similar. If this is not done, the mind will be prejudiced in spite of your best endeavors. I have to fight that with every fresh case I come to. I have to labor to keep myself from thinking about the things I have cured like that before, because it would prejudice my mind.

SUGGESTED STEPS FOR EXAMINING THE PATIENT AND CASE RECORDING

- *As we said, case - recording is an art and one has to observe all the preliminaries including interrogation, inspection, palpation, percussion, auscultation and special examination of the patient recording the name, age, gender, profession, and disease history.*

- Let the patient narrate his or her complaints. Write down the complaints turn by turn and leave some space between each complaint so that you can write further on that particular complaint when you want an answer later.
- Write the complaints right from beginning to the day of patient's coming to you i.e. make a sequence.
- After you have written the history as above, now pay attention to the constitutional make-up of the patient. These are of three types, the structure of the patient, the mental make-up or emotional state and place of living (damp house, hilly terrain, ill-ventilated house etc.)
- Enquire about the family history of patient like tuberculosis, asthma, rheumatism, cancer, epilepsy, diabetic, cardiac problems etc.
- Now come to the physical examination. Check the pulse, temperature, respiration, inability to sit or stand for a long time etc.
- Start checking from the head downwards. The patient's face will tell the mental condition as to whether he or she is worried, angry, depressed or frustrated. Note if there are black spots beneath the eyes or much below the facial line, yellowness of eyes, whitish skin of face, having long sighs by the patient with the result of inflation of nasal cavity, wrinkles on the forehead; ulcers, eruptions, pustules on the face.
- Inspect the goiter, if any, feel the carotid pulsation, dilatation of the veins, any skin disease on the neck and glands, sepsis of the mouth, emaciation etc.
- See the chest and back for any rickets (children) or emphysema (here the chest is protruded outside). Place your hand on the chest or back spreading it here and there to locate any bony change or pathological change. Ribs and clavicles must be checked for any inflammation or tumor etc.

- Now go in for percussion. Place your middle finger of the left-hand on the chest or back of the patient and tap the finger with the help of your right hand index fingertip. The resonance will give a different sound of vibrations, dullness etc. It is a clue towards the condition of lungs. The tapping would be systematically. First, tap the upper part right side of the chest and then the left side. Similarly, tap the parts in the middle part of chest, right and left and finally the lower part of the chest, right and left.
- Now with the help of stethoscope, check the heart and lungs. The lungs need the same systematical examining i.e. upper, middle and lower part of the chest or back, both right and left.
- X-ray and laboratory tests as needed are additional assets.

We should agree that a part of the above examination is for the allopathic nature of complaints. The examination gives us a little knowledge about the disease so far as homoeopathic treatment is concerned. Now we come to the questionnaire for the doctor. He should put the following questions:

- What are the foods that aggravate the condition? What about appetite, thirst, liking of salt or sugar etc., cravings and aversions?
- What about tiredness, sleeplessness, restlessness, dreams, peculiar trends during sleep, wants to keep the body covered or wants windows open etc.?
- What about sexual desires, aversions and any peculiar obsessions about sex-acts?
- What about emotions, phobia, fears, anxiety, concentration of mind, forgetfulness, delusions, mental symptoms and memory etc.?
- What about menstrual functions, birth of babies, abortions, leucorrhoea and pain in the uterus region?

- What about the various systems of body including stomach, abdomen or liver disorders, nature of urine, stool and associated complaints, burning of extremities, sweating, skin eruptions, drandruff, joint pains, respiratory problems, and endocrine or circulatory disorders?
- What about the condition of health and its changes during day or night or any particular season?

All the above questions *should not be put directly* to the patient but make your questions in such way that *they appear indirect*. Let the patient tell his suffering on his own. For example, if the condition about menses is to be enquired, simply ask, what about the menses? Never say, "Are your menses profuse, scanty, irregular and so on?" Just say, "How about menses?" In all cases, such questions should be avoided which have a simple answer, yes or no.

THE SECOND PRESCRIPTION

Once the homoeopathic medicine has been given and some results have been noted, it is better to evaluate the same for the second prescription. For this, note the changes in the appetite of the patient, digestion, stool habit, skin eruptions, cycle of menstruation, sexual urge and mental state. Such changes lead to correct sound remedy or change in the potency of the remedy. There are many types of patients. Some will come and report that after taking your homoeopathic medicines, his or her palms and soles have started burning. Now have a check on the past history of the patient, whether he/she had the problem before taking allopathic drugs. If it has returned, you are on the right path. Consider the same medicine on a higher potency level or think of a complementary to see the results, which will be positively be on the amelioration side. If there are some new complaints upon taking the homoeopathic remedy, note these and change the prescription according to the new symptoms. If the patient feels no change in his/her condition after taking homoeopathic medicine but the patient reports 'feeling good or general well-being feeling', the doctor should think that he is on the right path. There is no need for changing the prescription, even placebo can be recommended.

THYROID PROBLEMS — A MIASMATIC STUDY

The greatest asset to the era of Homoeopathy lies with the conception of miasmatic theory initiated by the great master, Hahnemann. Miasmatic theory has no connection with the chemical and mechanical activities or force of the body. This is the theory of an invisible vital force without which there would not be any organic chemistry. Hahnemann understood the wrong conception of the times in respect of medicines and revolted against it. He neglected all the prevailing systems declaring them unscientific. According to him, the spring could not reach a higher level than the source. This is really true. Hahnemann reached the spring source and proved that the allopathic medicine system cannot reach the height of the spring i.e. homoeopathy. Now when we see back and watch the progress made by both the systems, we find that the allopathic system has not changed materially and that their modes and methods of procedure have changed. The allopathy has abandoned certain old values and methods and accepted new ways, which are also with certain drawbacks of side effect etc. On the other hand, homoeopathy sails in the same boat having the same principles but with a refined outlook. Now allopaths do agree to send their patients to the homoeopaths, for treatment of warts, skin diseases and removal of kidney stones without operation. What I am pointing out is that a system without a law cannot be compared with a system having a fixed law.

Why a miasmatic study is required for treatment in Homoeopathy is standing question among the learners? I quote here J.H. Allen from his book, 'Chronic Miasms and Pseudo Psora'

(B. Jain Publishers, 1994) for a better understanding of the theory of miasms.

"Someone may ask, why it is necessary for a true homoeopath to know about these chronic miasms as long as he prescribes according to the law of similars and cures the cases. There are many reasons why he should be able to distinguish their presence in the organism, whether it is psora, latent syphilis, especially the tubercular form, or whether it be sycosis. Dr. Hering, however, in his introductory remarks in the Organon (3rd American edition) thinks it not of vital importance: What important influence can it exert whether a homoeopath adopts the theoretical opinions of Hahnemann or not, so long as he holds the principal tools of the master and the materia medica of our schools? What influence can it have, whether a physician adopt or reject the psoric theory as long as he selects the most similar medicine possible."

The fact is that we cannot select the most similar remedy unless we understand the phenomena of the acting and the basic miasms, whether we are conscious or unconscious of the fact. The curative remedy is but the pathopoesis of a certain pathogenesis of an existing miasm. The proving of the remedy would be very indefinite to us if the name were withheld from us. Suppose that you were making a proving of *Sulphur* or *Aconite*. Why, the first thing you would do, would be to ask for their names, you would say, I shall not attempt to use these remedies without knowing their names. So, it should be with the disease-producing agent. We should know, not only the name of that underlying principle that fathers that phenomena with which we are so diligently and earnestly contending and combating. It is the difference between an intelligent warfare and fighting in the dark; it is no longer a battle in the mist. Again, suppose we prescribe the similar remedy and have no knowledge of the law of action and reaction (or Primary and Secondary action) how can we watch the progress of a case without a definite knowledge of these disease forces (miasms), with their mysterious but persistent progressions, pauses, rests, forward movements, retreats, and attacks among unfamiliar lines, and of whose multiplied modes of action we have taken no cognisanse? In fact when we know nothing about the traits and characteristics of our enemy, is it possible to wage an equal warfare? Suppose that one would say that disease was due to bacteria, to a certain germ, to atmospheric conditions, to taking cold—facts to which the majority of diseases are attributed, would those facts assist us in the selection of the similar remedy? Would they help us to understand the phenomena of germ development, of taking cold? Why should he take a cold? Why should disease return in the same form or some diverse form? These are the things that disturbed the mind of Hahnemann, and landed him to discover the psoric theory of the disease."

According to Allen, the doctors who select the similar remedies to cure their patients are not true healers of the sick because they are ignorant of the causes and effects of the disease.

IMPORTANCE OF KNOWING THE MIASMATIC THEORY

In Aphorism 15 of the Organon, Hahnemann describes his theory of miasms, "The suffering of the immaterial vital principle which animates the interior of our bodies, when it is morbidly disturbed, produces symptoms in the organism that are manifest" and it is these morbidly produced symptoms that constitute what is known as disease in all multiplied forms, whether functional or structural. Knowledge of all miasmatic theory is complete knowledge of all that is known as disease, and beyond these symptoms there is nothing discoverable or recognizable as disease. This, Hahnemann elaborates in Aphorism 19 of Organon: "Disease is nothing more than changes in the general state of the human economy, which declare themselves as symptoms."

This also means that disease is the aftereffect (influence) of some subversive force, acting in conjunction with the vital force, subverting the action and changing the physiological momentum. *Here, Allen is again referred for his philosophical definition of disease, "Disease is the totality of the effects, by which we recognize or perceive the action of a peculiar order of subversive forces upon an organism which has been exceptionally or specially adapted to, or prepared for their reception."*

This statement makes the theory of miasms more clear. A close study of the above statement draws a conclusion that disease is the vicarious embodiment of some miasmatic influence that has bonded itself with the life force, producing disease according to the type, as is seen in psora or any other of the chronic miasms.

It has been seen that a well-selected remedy given for the symptoms totally cures the case for time being. The symptoms are removed but after sometime, they return with same or more firmer force. This means that the disease has some deep roots in the body of the sufferer. The disease had been removed temporarily with the use of higher potency medicine but this time the return is with some change in expression of the symptoms. Most of the time, these changes point to the order of the disease in the earlier stage. A man having a skin disorder gets cured but his earlier disease, asthma returns. When asthma is cured, his severe backache returns. What does all this show? What is source of the existence of the disease? It must be some latent, inherent, internal, pre-existing cause, having its habitat in the organism. Such habitat is not connected with the material body but with the dynamism or the life force. Thus it becomes a part of life force. We spoke of skin disease. Skin does not produce an eruption by itself, (leave aside the mechanical or chemical or traumatic reasons) and does not get a morbid state unless it is obliged by some previous perverted change of abnormal activity in the organism itself. An eruption is an expression that the disease inside has come out. The disease from a latent stage is now living and it certainly has a background of miasms through which its opening had been possible. The background is psora here.

THE THREE MIASMS

After twelve years of deep study on the patients, Hahnemann concluded that there are three basic miasms, which are the underlying causes of all chronic diseases. Further, he pointed out that a patient may be a victim of one miasm or may have combination of miasms. As we discussed earlier, the first one is psora miasm. *'Psora'* derived from Greek language means *itch*. As per Hahnemann, this is the earliest miasm affecting the mankind or human race with the most fundamental hidden element of debility or disease. It is the underlying debility, which gives rise to various other diseases. Hahnemann made a related history or link of diseases like diabetes, arthritis, cancer, mental diseases, epilepsy etc. with *psora*.

The second miasm in the row is *syphilitic* miasm with which the human race is affected. The name of the disease, 'syphilis' is considered to be one of the manifestations of this miasm. Besides this disease, there is a wide range of other disorders attached with the miasm. Hahnemann had formed an idea that those who suffered from syphilis miasm acquired this disease through exposure to the basic disease, syphilis or it might have been by inheritance from an infected ancestor. This miasm runs from family to family of generations.

The third miasm discovered by Hahnemann was the *sycosis* miasm. In Greek language, *syco* means *fig*. It is the manifestation of the disease gonorrhea whether contacted by the patient or by one of the patient's ancestors.

On combinations of the miasms. Hahnemann is very clear and cites an example. If a person is weakened by the psora miasm but is also exposed to venereal diseases by one of his or her sins or sexual conduct, he or she is bound to be sick with the second miasm. This combination then runs from generation to generation.

Can we say with authority that such and such disease by name is the outcome of psora, syphilis or sycotic miasm? No, we cannot say so because of severe intermingling of miasms at different stages of the disease. Let us see. *We consider psora miasm responsible for itch or eczema, syphilitic miasm exhibits ulcers and sycotic miasm, a disease of figs (skin disease)* but this is proved that all three miasms can result in any pathological change. Cancer, diabetes, insanity or imbecility can arise from the last stage of any of the miasms or from any combination of them.

THE MIASM BEHIND THYROID DISEASES

With this explanation of miasm, we come to our subject. Thyroid disease has many faces of symptoms. Behind this disease, lies a disease process that is set up in the infected organism before a local or constitutional disease manifests itself to the senses of the patient or the observer (doctor). Psora is considered as the miasm of the human civilization and is responsible for $7/8^{th}$ of human diseases. Psora, therefore, cannot be disconnected from the thyroid diseases, the symptoms of which are many. At the same time, this disease has links with syphilis and sycosis. We have already considered in our chapter of therapeutics that iodine is one of the main remedies for thyroid diseases. Have a thorough examination of this remedy in terms of miasmatic angle.

"*Iodine meets all the miasms, and especially the tubercular and syphilitic.* The menses are premature, copious and the patient suffers much during the flow. It may also be too late or retarded. When delayed, the patient suffers from severe vertigo and palpitation of the heart. The flow is unusually acrid; it excoriates the thighs and is followed by an acrid, slimy leucorrhea. The patient is hungry during the menses...and so on," says J.H. Allen in chronic miasms.

Lyc. is another remedy which has been found useful in thyroid diseases. *Lyc.* is a powerful *anti-sycotic*, deep in action and cures almost any state of miasmatic state of system even to a mixed miasm or malignancy.

Natrium muriaticum is also stated to be a good remedy for thyroid diseases and it is wonderful to note that this remedy is *pseudo-psoric*.

Bromium supposed to be good remedy for thyroid disease is also *pseudo-psoric*.

Calc. has a marked *pseudo-psoric* trait if its chronic gonorrhea is taken into account. It is also a great *anti-psoric* like *Sulphur*.

Where does all this explanation of main remedies lead us to? To which miasm? Well, it is not easy to point to a single miasm responsible for thyroid diseases. Hahnemann himself says that disease is a disturbance of the life force. We know very little about this life force even after two hundred and fifty years of the era of Hahnemann. According to different scholars of homoeopathy, the disease of thyroid cannot be attributed to psora, pseudo-psora, sycosis, syphilis or combinations of these great central distributors of life. It is difficult to classify this disease with one or more of miasms because the symptoms sometimes point to one miasm at the beginning and go to other miasm in the middle of disease and end in another miasm eventually.

As a matter of fact, the disease of thyroid has many layers of predisposition, which go through the phases of waxing and waning of temporary ailments from time to time. These are always taken into account while treating the cases of thyroid in homoeopathy. The prescriber or the doctor has to systematically remove layer upon layer of predisposition in respect of debility or disease, step by step according to symptoms produced in the body. Each layer once removed will bring the next set of symptoms and a change in prescription should be made to remove the existing layer. Such a case is always of chronic nature. Suppose *Sulphur* has been given and *Lyc.* is the next remedy selected, the prescriber has to examine whether the intermediate remedy *Calc.* suits or not. The general rule applies here and it will always be better to give a dose of *Calc.* before *Lyc.* is given.

Finally, when we examine all the discussion as above, it can be concluded that the diseases of thyroid belongs to psora and sycosis miasms in general. These are major influences observed in daily practice. However, it is also to be kept in mind that each prescription has to be based upon the totality of symptoms at the moment.

Thyroid disease is the outcome of an exciting cause, which in turn goes on increasing if not treated properly. By 'properly', I mean by homoeopathy. The patient of thyroid disease is mostly on allopathic drugs when he comes to a homoeopath. So, exciting cause has already become a maintaining cause by dint of allopathic drugs. This is what we think. The surprising fact is that we hold allopathic drugs responsible for maintaining cause, which is not so in total. It may be true partially. The actual reason behind the maintaining cause is the inherited chronic disease predisposition i.e. miasm. The predisposition generated by the parents is the result of state of the health, which goes from generation to generation.

MOST SUITABLE MEDICINES

Important antipsoric medicines

Alum., Aloe, Amb., Anac., Ant-c., Apis, Arg-n., Ars., Ars-i., Aur., Bar-c., Bell., Benz., Berb., Borx, Bufo, Calcarea group of medicines, Carbons, Cap., Ferrum group of medicines, Kali group, Lach., Led., Lac-c., Lyc., Magnesia group, Natrium group, Acid nitric, Petr., Phos., and its acid, Plat., Plb., Psor., Pyrog., Sil., Sep., Sar., Sec., Sel., Stann., Staph., Sulph., Sul-ac., Tarent.

Important anti-sycotic medicines

Arg-m., Arg-n., Benz., Berb., Calc-ars., Ars., Caust., Clem., Colch., Dulc., Ac-fluor., Iod., Kali bi., Kali c., Kali i., Lyc., Mag-c.,

Mag-m., Mag-p., med., mez., Mur-ac., Nat-ars., Nat-c., Nat-m., Nat-s., Nit-ac., Phos-ac., Phos., Psor., Pyrog., Sars., Sep., Sil., Staph., Thuj., Tub.

Important anti-syphilitic medicines

As we have said that the thyroid disease is limited generally to psora and sycosis miasm but there is no limitations or boundaries for any disease and hence given below are some important medicines belonging to anti-syphilitic group.

Ars., Ars-i., Aur-m., Calc-a., Fl-ac., Hep., Kali-bi., Kali-c., Kali-i., Lach., Lyc., Merc., Nit-ac., Phyt., Sars., Staph., Tub.

Please note that many of the medicines are useful in all the three miasms.

ENDOCRINOLOGY WITH REFERENCE TO THYROID PROBLEMS

We cannot ignore the fact that most of the human body problems have some trace of dysfunctions of glandular system. The thyroid problems including hypothyroid or hyperthyroid, goiter and other related manifestations are the result of endocrine imbalance. This is one view besides the one that we discussed above (miasms). We cannot forget the miasms in relation to the ailments, be they endocrine or otherwise because we do not consider a human body in compartments like allopathy where a general physician will send the patient to a specialist. We consider that the human being is a unit, mind, body and spirit and they are so inter-related or correlated as to act freely and without impediment, when the vital force is in equilibrium. When this equilibrium is imbalanced due to some exciting or maintaining cause, the whole unit of body is affected to a greater or less degree. Having this type of concept in mind there is no doubt that there is a great importance of endocrine glands in maintaining our health, especially when we know that it is the infinitesimal amount of glandular secretion, which is responsible for a bright upkeep of the body in true sense. Thyroid and its associated helping glands prove the fact that health has a deep bearing with these secretions in proper amount with proper timing and age.

ENDOCRINOLOGY NOW WELL KNOWN TO HOMOEOPATH

There is an interesting discussion on the fundamentals of endocrinology in the book named, 'Endocrinology' written by August A. Werner (Lea and Febiger, 1937). Let us see how we can gain our knowledge from it so far as thyroid is concerned.

"There has been much complaint from physicians in general that the literature on endocrinology is technical and difficult to understand. There are several reason for these seeming difficulties, among which may be mentioned the newness of the subject; the lack of definite information as to the possible number of hormones and their functions; the intricate inter-relationship of the secretions of the ductless glands; the difficulty in application of the results of animal experimentation to the human, which, aside from the scientific value of such work, is the ultimate object of these investigations; the variation of potency of the hormonal preparations used, and the difficulty of determining the individual dosage, which is influenced by the degree of function of the glands of the patient, the individual susceptibilities of the patient, cellular receptivity, interaction of other endocrine secretions, and the effect of general metabolic factors and disease processes in each individual.

To be a good clinical endocrinologist, one must first be a good internist, and the time is not far distant when, in order to be a good internist, one must be a good endocrinologist.

It is necessary to have:

1. A thorough knowledge of the anatomical structure and

arrangement of the autonomic nervous system. Its division into two parts, viz. the parasympathetic and the sympathetic; knowledge of the function of these two divisions that are diametrically opposed to each other when stimulated.

2. Comprehension of the function of the endocrine glands; so far as this has been definitely or reasonably established.

3. The recognition that the intricate vital life processes of the body over which we have no control, such as the regulation of normal growth and development, the digestion, the absorption, and assimilation of food and its release from the storehouses, such as the liver and muscles for the production of energy, the continuation of cardiac action and respiration at a normal rate. Our sense of well being; all these and more, depend in great measure upon the maintenance of delicate equilibrium between the two divisions of the autonomic nervous system.

4. A knowledge that the maintenance of this functional balance between the parasympathetic and sympathetic divisions of the autonomic nervous system is markedly influenced by the internal secretions of the ductless glands which act as governors over it......"

"There is a great clamor from the medical profession for the information on treatment of endocrine conditions. Before we can treat any abnormal condition successfully we must first have knowledge of the syndrome and its etiology and secondly, we must have potent preparations for treatment. Many endocrine syndromes have been recognized in the past before active principles were available for treatment. This condition still exists and the possession of active hormones does not always ensure that relief can be given for obvious reasons. With the desire and urge to alleviate these endocrine syndromes, all manner of glandular preparations have been utilized, many of which are inert, especially when administered orally......"

This above reference has been given by Herbert A. Roberts in his book 'The Principles and Art of Cure by Homoeopathy' (B. Jain Publishers, 1995) and we must take a note that the above narration is very much related to thyroid gland. Coming back to the modern times from the reference, it is well known that our students of BHMS have a thorough knowledge of physiology, anatomy and internal hormonal diseases of the glands. They know the fundamentals of endocrinolgy although they have no specialization in this subject. Knowing the fundamentals is enough and making a systematic case history of the patient in respect of symptoms can solve thyroid diseases.

There is very little doubt that the majority of cases of under or over-development of tissues or organs (obesity, inhibition of or precocious development of sex characteristics traceable to pituitary, pineal or thyroid glands or the gonads) and variable skeleton formations (for instance dysfunction of the parathyroid) are all *manifestations of miasms*. This confirms our theory of miasms as we have discussed in the last chapter. According to our great master, this may be outcome of either inherited or acquired. In India, while dealing with the cases of thyroid diseases, it has not been established whether the patients had any family history. At least this has been my personal experience. The reason behind this strategy is that the people did not know the name of the disease and also could not tell whether their parents or maternal or paternal side of family had this disease. The disease had an established character only after fifties, that too in affluent classes. The only disease related to the neck and known to the people was *goiter*.

Be it hereditary or acquired, there is no doubt that the orthodox school believes in the objective symptoms supported by the values of thyroid function test but the homoeopathic school gives importance to the individual's subjective manifestations in accordance with Hahnemann's logical development of the therapeutic principle. The best part of this therapy is that today homoeopathy is also supported by laboratory and other functional tests and it is more jeweled by our rich worth of materia medica and homoeopathic philosophy. Besides these tools, we have our repertories, constitutional symptoms, mental and physical symptoms, peculiar and individual symptoms to bring forth the remedy having corresponding values. We have, therefore, reasonable possibility of cure in the thyroid diseases.

NEED FOR RESEARCH AND PROVING OF MEDICINES

Coming back to Roberts, who has given a wealth of arguments on endocrinology in his above referred book makes a comment on the need for finding out more remedies to combat the diseases. For this, he has referred to the editorial in the October 1938 issue of the *British Homoeopathic Journal*.

"In estimating the possibility of successful homoeopathic treatment of deficiency diseases we must, of course, recognize that the action of drugs is by eliciting a response from a living cell; they cannot do this from those that are dead or restore them to life. It is of no use to attempt the impossible. But we should also recognize that no organ or tissue becomes suddenly destroyed, unless it be by trauma, and that there are all degrees of failure of function, and if the failure has not gone too far it should be, and we believe it is possible to restore it to the normal by giving the simillimum. To this end we need a deeper acquaintance with our remedies. We are using practically the same materia medica that we did fifty or more years ago. It required no alteration, but it does need to be added to, not by the addition of more remedies but by the fresh proving to pursue the action of drugs into the realm of modern physiological research, and especially their action on the endocrine organs. If we do not increase our knowledge of the capabilities of our drugs our homoeopathic art will become static. It will make no progress."

WHY NOT GO AGAINST THE CURRENT TO SEE NEW RESULTS?

This is very much true even today. We have same materia medicas (most popular—Boericke), same repertories (mostly Kent and Boenninghausen) which suggest familiar rubrics. The students along with practicing doctors make use of the same remedies without addition of new proved remedies. Check on the other side of the picture, the symptoms of the patients have changed even for those proved remedies because of the changed environment and changed food habits added with highest level of pollutions. How can the Homoeopaths be mentally satisfied or justify with the aggravation of *Lyc.* having a trait of 4 to 8 P.M. or with the aggravation of *Ant-t.* in spring, dampness, and cold weather when the timing, seasons and thermal conditions were not subjected to Indian climate and conditions. *Ant-t.* is being given in all the seasons of the year in India and I have not observed any ill-effects of this remedy. It is matter of imposed belief through books that we in India still continue to give the remedies in the fashion written in the books and do not venture to deviate from the course or go against the current. There are very few homoeopaths who have really experimented on this aspect. I have been giving *Lyc.* to the patients and never instructed them to avoid its intake between its aggravation times (4-8 P.M.). When the remedy has an aggravation at a particular time and there is same aggravation time in symptoms of the patient, there is every reason to use the remedy, be its induction at any time. In no rational thinking, one is prevented to induct the remedy during the time of aggravation. Find it yourself and you will be surprised that *Lyc.* will not prove useless or aggravate the condition of the patient if given between 4 to 8 P.M., provided the patient has all the symptoms of *Lyc.*

This way by experimentation only we can find a new trait of the remedy but who dares to do it for want of professional benefits? But those who do it are also not exposing their result to fellow homoeopaths. How can homoeopathy advance if such is the behavior of fellow learners? Homoeopathy can only make advancement when the result of particular cases and traits of medicines are exposed through literature.

If you happen to screen the bookshops dealing in homoeopathic literature, you will be surprised that not many books on thyroid diseases are available.

Recently I went through an article on thyroid gland in Times of India dated 8th September, 2002 wherein the author has mentioned following remarks in favour of homoeopathy.

"Homoeopathy is absolutely remarkable in treating thyroid dysfunction......"

There is certainly some reason why such a compliment has been given to Homoeopathy. It is the outcome of a series of research work by the author of the article or the doctor who has been referred to in the said article. There are homoeopaths who make experiments and make them known as well for the public but they can be counted on fingers. There is no speciality cadre given to the Homoeopaths as in the case of Allopathy but the time is no far when the present generation, doing M.D. in Homoeopathic subjects, would display specialization against their names. It is also said that there is no R & D in Homoeopathy. This is not true. The ministry of Health and Family Welfare, with the help of ISM & H (Indian System of Medicine and Homoeopathy) has separate department to promote Homoeopathy and make research, efforts are being made and many big companies dealing with manufacture of Homoeopathic medicines are trying to integrate the ongoing R & D with homoeopathic medicines.

When we talk of research and development, it is not that people are not aware of the development and drawbacks of allopathy. As a matter of fact, people are now drawn towards alternative system of medicines. Dr. Mosaraf Ali and Dr. Issac, practitioners of modern medicines have worked a lot on alternative therapies. They have pioneered a new system of intergrated medicines in which number of alternative therapies can be given at a time. Dr. Ali has written a book 'The Integrated Health Bible' in which he explains how all the systems of medicines can be used without adverse effects. Dr. P.E. Abraham, MD, of Bangalore turned to alternative medicine like homoeopathy, yoga, ayurveda and is of the opinion that doctor's role is to initiate the healing process, and if other procedures can help, they should be welcome. The pattern of thinking is changing. The doctors belonging to all disciplines have to be open-minded and will have to believe in the systems other than they practice. Let us hope so, at least for the betterment of humanity.

On thyroid diseases, there is lot to be done to eliminate the orthodox pattern for which the patient is also not in favor. The patient is fed up with daily intake of orthodox medicine and it is the time when homoeopathy or other systems of medicines can click provided due attention is given to the experimentation in respect of atleast thermal conditions (aggravations, ameliorations etc.), if not all the modalities. This is a field where homoeopaths can do a remarkably good work.

■

Should Allopathic Medicine be Stopped

STOPPING INTAKE of allopathic medicine by the patient of thyroid disease and starting directly homoeopathic medicine in its place is not at all advised. The complications involved in such a procedure have to be understood first. The daily intake of a tablet of allopathic medicine for years is bound to affect the particular symptoms, the body had before this medicine was started. Now what we see and find out from the patient are the symptoms produced by the continuous intake of this medicine. Suppose a patient had restlessness and anxiety post afternoon before intake of this allopathic medicine, our homoeopathic medicines would have been *Anac., Bry., Chin., Lach., Phos., Puls., Staph.,* and *Sulph.* (Reference: Boenninghausen's Therapeutic Pocket Book). But now, after continuous intake of Eltroxin, the restlessness is gone or we should say there is suppression of actual symptoms. This was the symptom, which was consistent throughout the history of the patient when his thyroid problem started. What we conclude is that the symptoms at present cannot be evaluated as true and that the body's defense mechanism has also changed due to continuous use of drug.

So, what is the course of action now? Yes, we select a remedy according to the present symptoms and give it in lower potency with rapid frequency and watch the results. Along with this remedy of homoeopathic system of medicine, Eltroxin has to be continued because *its discontinuation may stir and imbalance the defense mechanism of the body*. If the remedy given by homoeopath is based upon totality of symptoms and simillimum, there are bound to be good results. At this juncture, the allopathic drug has to be decreased in the fashion suggested in the following paragraphs. In no case, the patient should be made to understand that there would be drastical favourable changes upon decreasing the frequency of allopathic drugs. Sometimes, there may be a relapse and then again allopathic drug has to be started.

This type of treatment needs a high degree of skill in both allopathic and homoeopathic handling of the case. The body has to be given some time to return to normal and at a position when so called suppression took place. There is no doubt that the defense mechanism of the body will react upon use of homoeopathic medicines and what is needed is patience by the patient and use of utmost skill by the homoeopath.

Once the patient is satisfied on the above aspect and homoeopathy appeals to him, it becomes easier for the practitioner to go ahead with his treatment. One thing is important here that the patient must be told to have patience and give some time for the treatment as we said earlier. The very fact that the patient is ready to take orthodox medicine for his lifetime gives homoeopathic system a boost. You will find your patient to wait and watch when getting treated in homoeopathy. He will give you enough of time and now it is your duty to select his remedies carefully. It is your skill now to monitor the progress. It has to be made clear here that the medicine of the orthodox system should not be stopped immediately and this should be continued along homoeopathic medicines for considerable time so that homoeopathy finds its root into the system of the body. When the relief in some symptoms is observed, the allopathic medicine should be taken on alternate days instead of taking daily. Please note that the relief will be in some symptoms, which were continuously present and not eliminated even during the intake of allopathic medicines for years. This is a sure sign of effect of homoeopathy. When this occurs, the homoeopath develops a confidence that his selection of medicine is bearing fruits. He can then proceed ahead by selecting further remedies to eliminate other symptoms. This may take months together but once this stage is achieved, the homoeopath can tell the patient to stop intake of orthodox medicine in the following manner.

THE SUGGESTED COURSE OF HOMOEOPATHIC AND ALLOPATHIC MEDICINES

- Elimination of a single symptom from the body means that the intake of allopathic medicine can now be done on alternate days.
- Now watch whether the symptom removed has returned or permanently gone and the patient feels any discomfort.
- Has any new symptom come up? If so, give the symptomatic homoeopathic medicine to remove the new symptom.
- If the new symptoms does not get eliminated in spite of giving a homoeopathic remedy, allow the patient to resume the intake of his allopathic remedy daily instead of alternate day doses.
- Now select a different remedy basing upon constitution or basing upon miasm and watch. It is the selection of remedy that is at fault i.e. the physician is at fault and not the remedy.
- Upon a review in selection of remedy, the new symptom has to get eliminated. Once it is done, again advise the patient to move his alternate day intake therapy of his allopathic medicine.
- Coming back to the old state when a symptom was removed initially, now give remedy for the other symptoms. Upon this, when the other one or two basic symptoms are removed by homoeopathic medicines, it is time to reduce the intake or

orthodox medicine. Now, tell the patient to take his allopathic medicine after every two days instead of alternate day.
- Again watch the patient's symptoms and proceed in the same manner as advised. Go on reducing the intake of orthodox medicine and bring it to weekly and then fortnightly and later monthly but go on giving your selected homoeopathic medicine in increased potency on intervals if it has suited. *Make use of plenty of placebo* in between the high potency period. Give enough time to the remedy to act so that it brings in quick favourable changes.
- After giving proper homoeopathic medicine, the monthly dose of orthodox medicine be stopped. Now continue with your medicine, be it placebo or otherwise, as per your judgment based upon the remnant symptoms.
- Finally you will find that the patient is cured of the disease and of course it is going to take enough of time.

Here I would like to quote *Dr. George Vithoulkas* on thyroid cases on the above subject of use of allopathic medicine and its connection with homoeopathy. These are particularly his views taken from his book 'The Science of Homoeopathy (B. Jain Publishers, 1998)

"Thyroid cases: Thyroxine is a drug which does not directly interfere with the action of the homoeopathic medicine, but it does mask the symptomatology which would lead to the correct remedy. It can be very difficult to find the remedy in such cases. The procedure used in this regard to corticosteroids should be followed here. Once the correct remedy is found, a time may come when the general health has improved sufficiently that thyroxine can be discontinued altogether." (Page 258)

On use of Eltroxin, there is another view expressed by *Dr. Farokh J. Master* in his book, 'The Bedside Organon of Medicine' (B. Jain Publishers, 1996).

"After thyroidectomy, I allow patients to use thyroxine tablets. However, for hypothyroidism, I allow Eltroxin, in the beginning stage. When you are treating a case of thyroid gland dysfunciton, thyroid function test every 6 months is essential." (Page 72)

CASE HISTORY OF A HYPOTHYROIDISM CASE

The patient coming to homoeopathy at the stages when they had already taken the conventional system medicines for years together are less likely to get relief sooner. Such cases are quite difficult to be cured. I agree that in my practice, I have not cured a single patient of hypo or hyperthyroidism of long standing—five to ten years or more. The cure is only possible when the patient has opted homoeopathy within three years of starting his treatment in allopathic regime. Moreover, a patient of thyroid diseases should have patience to continue the treatment in homoeopathy for a longer period of at least one year or so. This is every essential to cure the disease. Moreover, cases can be treated very effectively by homoeopathy provided the patient has faith in the system. I quote here a case of a Bengali woman of 36 years, living in Faridabad, who was referred to me after she was diagnosed as a case of hypothyroidism. She had started taking the medicine Eltroxin and was on it for about 5 months and feeling better as well. Her husband, a keen follower of homoeopathy, did not like her taking one tablet every morning and brought her to me. Since it is a very interesting case, it is my duty to state it in terms of treatment.

Mrs. K, age 36 years, has one son, 10 years of age. In appearance, she is obese and flabby. A confused personality with anxiety about health and fear of infectious diseases. She was unable to concentrate on one subject. Spoke very slowly and softly. Her feet and legs were swollen. The skin was dry. Her face looked swollen, dry and bulky. Thirst was normal. Constipation and flatulence at times when she took rich and fat food items, was the symptom she narrated. It was winter and she had complaints of cold feet for which she had only one alternative, not to remove socks even when going to bed. Pain in the lumber region was common when she stood more than an hour in the kitchen. She liked sweets, fish and eggs. Of course, this is common food liked by most of the Bengalis.

Thyroid function test showed a positive case of hypothyroidism and she had been prescribed Eltroxin, one tablet a day, which she had been taking religiously every morning.

Without going into any details about thyroid problem, the first thing to do in this case was to prescribe a remedy for her above physical problems, which showed a definite case of *Calc. Calc.* 200 which was given on tongue to be followed by S.L. on 1.3.01.

On 19.3.01, she reported that she had some aggravation of symptoms initially for three days but now feeling better. The edema of extremities was less, her constipation had gone and there was relief in the backache too. The patient was feeling better in all. S.L. was repeated for 15 days.

On 3.4.01, she was much better and now was the time to start her treatment for hypothyroidism. During the intake of *Calc.*, She was advised not to stop her daily intake of allopathic medicine for hypothyroidism. "*Thyroidinum* is supposed to be the leading remedy for hypothyroidism but it is not specific and it acts better in some forms and on some patients than other i.e. better upon sporadic than endemic cretinism." (George Royal, MD in his book Textbook of Homoeopathic Theory and Practice of Medicine – B. Jain Publishers).

The patient was given *Thyroidinum* 3x in tablet form, two tablets everyday for 15 days.

On 22.4.01, she came to the clinic and reported that she was feeling much better in all her symptoms. Her skin was not dry now (Was it due to change of weather or due to medicine?). Now she was told to take her dose of Eltroxin every alternate day instead of daily intake. Two tablets of *Thyroidinum* 3x were continued for another fifteen days.

On 10.5.01, she returned to the clinic feeling still better without taking her allopathic drug daily. *Thyroidinum* 3x was repeated and now she was told to take her allopathic medicine after every two days instead of alternate day as prescribed earlier by me.

On 26.5.01, the condition was same but she felt better inwardly. Now she was told to reduce her allopathic drug once a week. *Thyroidinum* 3x was continued in the same dosage i.e. BD.

She came back to the clinic on 13.7.01. She had continued *Thyroidinum* 3x twice daily after purchasing the same medicine from Kolkatta where she had gone in the mean time.

She was advised to go in for thyroid function test and it was found that her report was absolutely normal.

So it had taken more than four months to recover from hypothyroidism. The allopathic doctor who had prescribed her Eltroxin told her to stop the same as the test report was normal. The patient and her family are still under my treatment for other health problems from time to time.

■

Is There Any Prevention?

THE DISEASES can be avoided or prevented from occurring provided we know the reason for onset of the disease. We know the organic reason of thyroid malfunction but do not know the exciting reasons as we know in the case of infectious and bacterial diseases. We do not know why people develop these diseases. Take the case of goiter, the reason is known that it may be due to shortage or excess of iodine. In hilly terrains, we find this disease more common and claim that it is due to above reasons. How come that all the people living in the same area under same environment with same source of drinking-water, and same type of diet-nature do not get this disease. A member of a family gets it and not the whole family. The reason is not known and hence the experts in the conventional system of medicines claim that there is no sure way to prevent it. However, Homoeopath knows this dilemma. Naturally, the miasmatic causation acts here.

PREVENTION I— NO SMOKING

"Not smoking may help prevent it from developing or worsening" is the view of U.S.A. experts. According to it, people who smoke are about two times more likely to have Grave's disease and about seven times more likely to have Grave's ophthalmopathy than those who do not smoke."

We, homoeopaths, know why diseases occur in particular person in a family or why the diseases behave differently with every person. Not only the above diseases under discussions but all the diseases have an explanation in homoeopathy. We need not discuss about the theory of homoeopathy and vital force here but one thing is strange when we discuss about prevention. There is a great amount of controversy about prevention or prophylactics. There is reference of remedies in our materia medica and repertories and doctors have been giving these remedies to their patients. Is there any logic behind this when we religiously read the law of similars. If we study the law of similars, it has a simple statement that a remedy given to a healthy person is likely to produce the symptoms of the disease for which the remedy is indicated. This is what happened to our great Master Hahnemann when he took Cinchona bark. If this is the principle, where is the question of preventive? If I am healthy and I do not have any symptoms of hypothyroidism or any other disease but wish to be free of this disease, I should forget about the theory of using any preventive remedy in homoeopathy. When I do not have symptoms of disease, where is the question of taking any medicine and why to think of any prophylactic, even if it is written in the books?

Regarding 'no smoking' it is better logic to adopt good advice, be it related or not related to thyroid gland. We homoeopaths accept it and are free to advise our patients. No harm in doing so because we shall be making our society free of smoking habits.

PREVENTION II—NO ALCOHOL

Drinking alcohol in any form, let it be whisky, brandy, gin, rum or beer, is never thought to be good for health in any disease, why to speak of thyroid? However, with the trends of the modern day when people cannot avoid such borrowed habits from the present day culture, it has not been thought bad if someone drinks in a safe limit. A peg of whisky or a glass of beer is what can be said a safe limit. One good cultivated ritual in the women folks of India is that they do not drink liquor and they fear God and society if they do so. Women are the most wanted persons to get captured by thyroid diseases.

PREVENTION III—TAKING RECOMMENDED FOOD ITEMS

When the disease (goiter, hyperthyroidism or hypothyroidism) has set in and the patient is already on allopathic medication, he or she is not told to avoid certain food items or take some precautions. It is very common that the patient taking some allopathic medicine for thyroid or for heart becomes careless and takes the intake of medicine as routing. The patient, in such case, does not go to doctor for a check-up whenever there is some problem and increases the dose by himself. This is a funny procedure for life-long medication. But one should be careful and avoid certain food item.

Cabbage, turnip, cauliflower, sprouts or grams (dal), and spinach are to be avoided.

Reduce the saturated fats and replace them with monounsaturated and polyunsaturated fats. For this, the cooking oil medium has to be changed for the patient. Fat free oils are available in the market.

Patients with hyperthyroidism have high demand for nutrients. Vitamin B complex is one alternative if non-vegetarian food items like beef, pork, eggs, liver and vegetarian food items like cheese, full cream milk and potatoes are to be avoided. Those having overactive thyroid are prone to pernicious anaemia and hence taking vitamin B complex is essential for them.

Do not skip meals in any case because such a habit can lead to low blood sugar. With low blood sugar, the patient will feel tired, low of energy and would not feel like working.

INCLUDE THESE ITEMS IN YOUR DIET

- *Fresh fruits and vegetables* should be included in the diet everyday. At least three fruits should be included in the diet everyday.
- Take measured quantity of milk per day, say 150 ml, cheese, curds, eggs and items containing calcium. Food items like *soya beans, fish, peanuts, walnuts and green leafy vegetables should be included in the meals*. These items contain *calcium*, which is important for thyroid patients who are always at a risk to get osteoporosis. Calcitonin is one of the substances involved in regulating calcium levels in the blood and also it is one of the thyroid hormones.
- To help metabolize calcium, *magnesium* is also needed and for this, one should *take lemon, figs, grapefruit, sweet corn, almonds, apples and dark green vegetables*. Magnesium fights the depression and promotes healthier cardiovascular system.
- *Manganese* is another mineral, which is needed to help body manufacture thyroxine. It also helps remove fatigue, relax the muscles and improve the memory. Manganese is found in *green leafy vegetables, peas, beetroot, egg yolks and wholegrain cereals*.
- There is herb called Gotu Kol. In Sanskrit, it is named *brahmi*. Brahmi is stated to have derived from Sanskrit word Brahama, which means the whole universe, the Creator (God) of universe and all living beings, and the cosmic consciousness. If you look at the leaf of brahmi, it appears like two hemispheres of the brain. The herb helps flow of energy in the brain between the right and left hemispheres as per Ayurvedic System of Medicine. It has a definite action upon the brain, regulating hormones and producing higher consciousness. One-fourth teaspoonful of brahmi powder mixed with half teaspoonful of honey taken each morning helps cure thyroid diseases.
- Silver has very good healing powers for treating excessive 'pitta' (considering Ayurvedic theory for thyroid disease). Silver

promotes stamina and strength. Hyperactivity of thyroid gland can be somewhat controlled by use of silver. Make it a habit to drink a cup of milk at bed time. This milk should be heated in a silver container. It will bring good results.

PREVENTION IV—EXERCISE IN A BALANCED WAY

Exercise is one of the best tools for keeping our body fit and prevent our body from many diseases. In case of this disease, the patient may be weak in muscles and joints. There may be easy fatigue and breathlessness. Besides all this, there is a way to find a suitable exercise. The best one which has been tried on patients and found beneficial in both hypothyroidism and hyperthyroidism is the exercises of neck. This is very easy and there is no tired feeling or breathlessness while conducting this.

- Move your head slowly towards left and then towards right. Count these movements and make sure to move your neck ten times to the left and then ten times to the right.

- Now move your head slowly downwards so that the chin touches the chest and then move it upwards so that you see the roof of your house or the sky. Do it ten times to each direction.

- Now move your head sideways to the direction of shoulders. Do it ten times to each side.

- Make a clockwise rotation of the neck, starting from lowering the head and slowly raising it as the rotation is made. Make it three times and then switch over to anticlockwise direction in the same manner. This exercise may be tiresome for patients initially. So, start this by doing one rotation to each side.

Gentle activities like walking, swimming and *Yoga* can prove beneficial and all these exercises depend upon the type of physique, you possess. Consult a physiotherapist before starting any exercise, which tires you. The exercises mentioned here are general but every patient has different physical capability and hence this advice. One has to agree that exercise is very essential, be it mild, moderate or vigorous. It has a direct link with release of hormone like substances in the body (endorphins) by which we feel satisfied, calm and relaxed. If the exercise is done alone, it has less of impact. Doing exercise with a companion, say your husband or wife, has dual benefit. The benefit of gaining confidence and getting motivation are the assets for future health programs. Begin the exercise and by the time your schedule gets regular, you will feel stronger and more energetic.

PREVENTION V—POSITIVE THINKING

The patient has to be told about the pace of disease and that it is going to take some time before the same can be eliminated. So, a lot of confidence is needed on the part of the patient to believe that he or she has to overcome this disease. When the doctor tells the patient never to miss the tablet, how can a patient feel that he is going to be well or recover from the disease. There is no question of getting this feeling so far as the allopathic drug therapy continues. Here is the role of homoeopathy. We have already discussed the mode of treatment and how the patient has to reduce the quota of her or his medicine. With this theme in the mind of the patient, there is likelihood of building confidence. This feeling would come to the patient, once homoeopathic medicines make their presence felt. A sort of well-being has to be there if the remedy replacing allopathic medicine gets to work.

The patient is already on allopathic medicine and at the utmost bottom line so far as his or her confidence is concerned. Now there is no further bottom line or deterioration of his or her moral.

With induction of a change in the line of treatment and ample of assurances from the homoeopath and in sighting the feeling of goodness, the patient is not to see any more bottom line of his or her condition. It is bound to move higher for after the deep bottom or low, the graph goes up like mountain. When the reality of new situation hits, the patient grows upwards with self-esteem. A self-acquired honor for health he has achieved by changing food habits, doing exercise and eating healthy.

Think positive and the health will be yours.

PREVENTION VI—CONTROL OF EMOTIONS

If there is anything, which hurts and increases this disease most, it is the emotions. After all, thyroid gland has a direct breathing with the brains. It has to command the body in respect of all thermal changes. It is the generator of the body and bound to get all its directives through the brain. If brain has devised some internal method to cope with emotions and tension in one's life and it works too, there is no problem and no disease will occur due to after-effects of emotions and tensions, but it is very difficult at the time of crisis.

Depression, self-doubt, tension, anger, or a failure etc. is transition. They never remain stationary in the mind. Easy or difficult mobilizing of power to deal with these problems varies from person to person. Those who know this art are free from diseases and those who take time to adjust with the crisis get less of diseases. But those, who do not know to combat the emotions and surrender to them fall prey to serious diseases. This is not a new phenomenon.

One has to find out a way to avoid the crisis of mind. People adopt many methods to do so. They hit domestic articles, smash cushions, break utensils, jumps over mattress, tear the books, and do all sorts of things to melt away their anger. There are people who would not speak when anger and move out of home, sit near river or lakes and hurl stones in the rivers. They would rebuke themselves, talk themselves loudly and find out a solution. Some people cry, especially the ladies. They would weep, cry, shout and exhibit their anger just to find themselves cooled down after sometime. Such things are normal vents for emotions and do not bring in any diseases. *Thyroid patients* have to be careful and control their emotions. They should go easy on their emotions. They should not think that the crisis *should* have been dealt the way they thought was correct. They should think that the crisis could have been solved in the way, the other party felt proper even when the other party is at fault. Time will make a way to wrong or right . *The crisis or the moment of anger has to be subsided by replacing word, 'should' by word 'could'.*

Whenever in depression, take a brisk walk and it may clear up the depression. It has been found that clinically, depression has nothing to do with walking but experiments have suggested that walking can help remove even clinical depression. A study was made in USA on this theory—antidepressants act more quickly to eliminate depression but those who do not take the medicines and keep walking daily get relief although in a later stage. Depressed persons, who are not on medication and start daily exercise and walking, are less likely to relapse than those who take antidepressant drugs alone to get relief from depression. *Walking is a perfect exercise.*

PREVENTION VII—CONTROL OF ANGER

There is no one living in the world, which has not experienced the devil of anger. Knowing that anger is the reason behind many ills, people indulge into it and then repent too. Anger for a while and having capacity to control it in seconds is something normal but those who develop anger on every petty matter are more prone to diseases. Anger prompts the release of stress hormones, which raise the blood pressure and heart-beat. Excess of these stress-hormones can damage heart arteries and heart muscles causing irregular heat beating. This can constrict blood vessels, disrupt plaque and block the artery causing a heart attack. In many TV serials and films, you must have seen actors dying due to excessive anger. It can happen in real life too. Anger also harms the immune system to which our thyroid disease is related. It is also true that anger cannot be suppressed. Suppressing anger is just like putting your foot on the brakes while you are driving your vehicle. You wind up with friction in the body's motor, says an expert in the study of anger at the University of South Florida. Anger should not be suppressed but exposed in a mild way rather than engaging in rages of emotional outbursts or crying. Say your words gently and then manage to escape the situation. *Weep if you want but do not cry loudly. Weeping will make you easy.*

HOW TO MANAGE ANGER?

- Whenever you feel angry, count up to ten and go out for a walk.
- Question yourself as to what angered you? Was it important to get angry over the matter you were discussing? Was the situation appropriate to get angry? Could you avoid it? Think about these three questions. Such an evaluation of yourself may cool you down.
- On getting angry, go to the writing table and take out a writing pad. Write about your thoughts. Why did your anger arise? What is the solution according to you to solve your problem of your anger or worry? Write all this and you will find a way out.
- We also get angry on the behaviour of other people's laziness, rudeness, recklessness and slow work. Think, how are you concerned with these attitudes of the others. Do not distrust other people's motives. You have nothing to do with their

motives. Change your attitude. Choose an intelligent way how to behave with others and people will not make you angry.

■

Last word

POSITIVE THINKING is the best tool to use in any disease why just to speak of thyroidism. When you start treatment, it is better to follow the following:

- When you go to bed, remember god and thank for a good day you have spent, even if it had been a bad day, disease wise. Assure yourself that you have started medicines and you will feel better with the intake of this medicine.

- When you get up in the morning, thank God that you spent the night peacefully, even if the night was restless for you. Spread both palms before your eyes, rub both the palms vigorously and then place them on your face, cheeks. Feel the warmth of love of your hands. It is hands only, which make you 'Karamyog'. Do it three times.

- Now think that you have started taking medicine and that you are feeling much better than yesterday with this medicine, even if you are not feeling better. This is called positive thinking.

GOD BLESS YOU

Note: This book is most valuable for friends, readers, doctors and philosophers who firmly believe in the loyal following of the principles of great master S. Hahnemann.

Bibliography

Organon of medicine: S. Hahnemann
Chronic diseases: S. Hahnemann
Lectures on Homoeopathic Materia Medica: J.T. Kent
Repertory of Homoeopathic Materia Medica: J.T. Kent
Lectures on Homoeopathic philosophy: J.T. Kent
Book of Surgery: Baily and Love
Atlas of Anatomy: Trevor Weston
Human Anatomy and Physiology: V. Tatarino
Comparative Materia Medica and Therapeutics: N.C. Ghosh
Essentials of Homoeopathic Materia Medica and Pharmacy: W.A. Dewey
Essentials of Practice of Medicine: Balram Jana
Homoeopathic Theory and Practice of medicine: George Royal
Plain Talks on Materia Medica with Comparisons: Pierce Willard Ide
Materia Medica: Hering
Leaders in Homoeopathic Therapeutics: E.B. Nash
Materia Medica: Lippe
Select Your Remedy: R.B. Bishamber Das
Homoeopathic Prescriber: K.C. Bhanja
Bedside Prescriber: J.N. Shinghal
From Old Age to Youth: Sidhartalankar

Endocrinology: August A. Werner
Chronic Miasms and Pseudopsora: J.H. Allen
The Principal and Art of Cure by Homoeopathy: H.A. Roberts
Therapeutic Pocket Book: Boenninghausen
Science of Homoeopathy: George Vithoulkas
Bedside Organon of Medicine: Farokh J. Master
Bhojan Dwara Chikitsa: Ganesh Narain Chauhan
Homoeopathic Family Practice: Bhattacharya
Domestic Physician: Constantine Hering
Thyroid Problems: Pasty Westcott
Repertory of Homoeopathic Nosodes and Sarcodes: Berkley Squire
Practice of Medicine: F.W. Price
Practitioners Guide of Gall Bladder Stones and Kidney Stones: Shiv Dua
Oral Diseases: Shiv Dua

BJ
1588
.T9 1903